Praise for

29 Gifts

‑⌒‑ ‥

"*29 Gifts* is luminous, vivid and transformative. Reading and living its words will contribute to the world in mighty ways!"
—SARK, national bestselling author of
Succulent Wild Woman and creator, PlanetSark.com

"Cami's message echoes the truth that generosity of the heart is designed into the very fabric of our being. Reading *29 Gifts* makes it obvious that each one of us, right where we are, surrounded with exactly what we have, is a perfect vehicle of givingness. Her intimate story, and those of others, illuminate how the power of giving is where genuine healing, meaning, and happiness are found."
—MICHAEL BERNARD BECKWITH, author of
Spiritual Liberation: Fulfilling Your Soul's Potential

"In the African village, the relentless challenge of physical survival causes people to dig deep into the well of their psyches to offer gifts of the heart—to family, community, spirit. These are the simple gestures which flow over the barrenness of daily living and the lack of creature comforts. Cami and Mbali have joined forces to help us realize that the spirit of the village lives in the simplest of kind-hearted and well-intentioned gestures, wherever they are offered. The message of this book has never been more relevant, more needed, more valuable."
—MALIDOMA PATRICE SOMÉ, author of *Of Water and the Spirit*

"Walker's a plucky writer, and it's hard not to be inspired by her story . . . Can '29 Gifts' work? Well, at the very least, it makes you more aware of the good in your life, and it shifts the focus from yourself to others."
—*Boston Globe*

"The relative simplicity of the *29 Gifts* movement is refreshing . . .
A fantastic book."   —Blogcritics.org

"*29 Gifts* stands out among other 'inspirational' books because
Walker doesn't hold back. She describes her disease and symptoms
in vivid detail. And it's that bravery which makes the process ring
true. Following Walker's journey, one realizes that most of us give
many little gifts each day. But without the right mindset, they seem
like little tasks instead . . . Read all at once or at leisure, *29 Gifts* is
worth your time. Not only does it put a face on MS, it puts a face on
perceptions and the power of the mind to overcome adversity."
                                                         —*Deseret News*

"For those of us immersed in pity parties because things aren't going
our way, Cami's book offers a way to transform our lives and help the
people around us. The best part: It doesn't have to cost a dime."
                                                         —*Tampa Tribune*

"A poignant and insightful account of the transformative power of
acts of kindness."   —*Saginaw News*

"Walker turns what could have been a book about self-pity into a
great read . . . and a creative way to get on with life."
                                                         —*Library Journal*

"Walker's book gives new meaning to the phrase 'giving is better than receiving' . . . The lessons of *29 Gifts* are applicable to
everyone, healthy or not. It is an easy, enjoyable read—but more
importantly, it opens a reader's eyes to the ultimate gift: giving
to others."
                           —*Momentum* (the magazine of the National
                                        Multiple Sclerosis Society)

"Why not embrace the spirit of giving with your own 29 days of
kindness?"   —Oprah.com

29 Gifts

How a
Month of Giving
Can Change Your Life

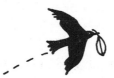

Cami Walker

You are
a gift!

Da Capo
∞
LIFE
LONG

A Member of the Perseus Books Group

Cami
Walker

Cataloging-in-Publication Data for this book is available from the Library of Congress.

HC ISBN 978-0-7382-1356-9
PB ISBN 978-0-7382-1430-6

First Da Capo Press edition 2009
First Da Capo Press paperback edition 2010

Published by Da Capo Press
A Member of the Perseus Books Group
www.dacapopress.com

Da Capo Press books are available at special discounts for bulk purchases in the U.S. by corporations, institutions, and other organizations. For more information, please contact the Special Markets Department at the Perseus Books Group, 2300 Chestnut Street, Suite 200, Philadelphia, PA 19103, or call (800) 810-4145 extension 5000, or e-mail special.markets@perseusbooks.com.

Editorial production by *Marra*thon Production Services
www.marrathon.net

DESIGN BY JANE RAESE
Set in 12 point Bulmer

10 9 8 7 6 5 4 3 2 1

This book is dedicated to
my mother and father, Carol and Larry Walker,
who taught me that the best way to solve
your problems is to help another person.

And to my husband, Mark Atherlay,
who held my hand through all of this.

You are all gifts.

Contents

II. Stories from the 29 Gifts Community

Prologue

Desperate Times, Desperate Measures

It is 4 a.m. and I am wide awake—again. I have not slept in sixty-three hours. Visions of myself crippled, unable to move my arms and legs, flash like red fire-exit signs in my mind. Thoughts spin uncontrollably, running in the same tired circles as I work myself into a full-fledged panic attack. Here I go again.

I'm going to end up in a wheelchair. I'll never be able to walk normally again. I'll never find a way to earn a living again. I'll never be able to write again. My friends and family will abandon me. My husband will get tired of taking care of me and leave me locked up alone in a nursing home before I'm 40, where I'll be ignored day after day and die before I'm 45 from infected bed sores.

I'll never get to be a mother.

Why have I been cursed with this horrible disease? Why can't the doctors cure multiple sclerosis . . . or at least give me some drugs that actually help? My life sucks. My life is over.

I want to die.

I try to lie quietly, not wanting to wake up Mark, my exhausted husband, who snores loudly beside me. *I can't believe that asshole can sleep while I'm having a nervous breakdown six inches away.*

I whimper and tears stream down my cheeks. My breath hitches, and I start to hyperventilate, causing Mark to stir in his sleep but not wake.

Just like when I was a child, my mother is keenly aware of my cries and comes to comfort me as soon as she hears me struggle. She is next door in our guest room, and I'm sure she has been lying awake worrying about me. She is staying with us for a while to relieve Mark, who is completely drained after several months of this daily drama.

My bedroom door cracks open, and I hear my mother's worried voice. "Honey, are you all right? Please try not to wake Mark. He's finally sleeping soundly. He's so tired."

"No," I hiccup softly. "I'm not all right." The words croak out of my throat, making a frog-like sound. It feels like an elephant is sitting on my chest. I can hardly speak but I manage to squeak out: "I'm scared."

My mother comes in and kneels down next to me, taking my left hand in hers. "I know you're scared, sweetheart. But everything is going to be okay," she reassures and reaches to switch on the lamp on the bedside table next to me.

"No, it's not!" I yell. The harsh words move the elephant from its resting place. I feel Mark startle awake and turn over in bed. My chest begins to heave and my cries increase in frequency. "I'm not okay! Nothing is okay! It's not going to be okay!"

Why can't they get it?

Mark's arms wrap around me from behind.

"Calm down, baby," he says softly in my ear. "You're getting yourself all worked up again. Take a deep breath and try to calm down."

Mark must be just as overwhelmed and frightened as I am, but he rarely raises his voice.

Just over two years ago, we took our wedding vows on a beautiful beach in Mexico. The photo stands next to the lamp by my bed. There we are, being showered in rose petals and holding hands. We look like we are in front of a fake prom backdrop, but the gorgeous blue sky and turquoise water behind us are real. As we looked out over the ocean, we believed there was nothing but clear skies ahead as we said, "I do," and pledged to support each other in sickness and in health.

Who could have predicted that the sickness part would start less than one month later? We returned home from our honeymoon and our world immediately turned gray and stormy as my health took a nosedive. I woke up one day and my hands were weak, tingly, and painful. Then a few days later, I lost the vision in my right eye. I was rushed to a team of specialists and within a week, the diagnosis of multiple sclerosis was confirmed.

Multiple sclerosis is a chronic, progressive disease of the central nervous system (the brain, optic nerves, and spinal cord). It's an autoimmune disease, which means the body's immune system attacks healthy cells in the body. In the case of MS, the immune system attacks the *myelin,* a protective fatty layer surrounding the nerves. Think of it as insulation that keeps the nerves firing smoothly. These immune system attacks create lesions in the myelin sheath. I imagine little holes being eaten in my nerve linings that leave areas of raw, exposed nerve prone to misfiring. Each person living with MS experiences a different set of often debilitating symptoms, depending on which nerves are affected. There's no cure. All that most doctors can do is offer patients medication, rehabilitation, and coping skills. A promising stem-cell treatment is being tested and other research is underway, but for now, MS is a disease that must be managed, not cured.

Primary symptoms—those arising directly from damage to the myelin and nerve fibers—include fatigue. Fatigue is one of the most common symptoms of MS, occurring in about 80 percent of people. Fatigue can significantly interfere with a person's ability to function at home and at work and may be the most prominent symptom in a person who otherwise has minimal activity limitations.

Other primary symptoms can include numbness, problems with mobility, balance, and coordination, bladder and bowel dysfunction, vision loss, dizziness, vertigo, sexual dysfunction, pain, cognitive difficulty, depression, muscle spasticity, tremors, speech disorders like slurred speech and difficulty finding words when speaking, swallowing problems, headaches, hearing loss and seizures, and respiration and breathing problems. A frighteningly daunting list, but different people exhibit different symptoms.

There are secondary symptoms, too—complications from these primary symptoms. For example, anyone whose bladder function is affected may suffer from frequent urinary tract infections. Or if someone has a lot of trouble moving and walking, the inactivity can result in loss of muscle tone, muscle weakness, decreased bone density, and risk of fracture.

Neither Mark nor I signed up for this. We both feel cheated out of the life we planned together: the house we planned to buy, the children we wanted to have. Those feel like absurd dreams now, since all we can do is hold on to each other for dear life and hope to come out the other side with our relationship intact.

My mom opens the drawer in my nightstand and gazes down at the large collection of prescription pill bottles, which she spent twenty minutes labeling yesterday afternoon. Each bottle now wears a nametag across its cap—a piece of blue painter's tape with my mom's neat, kindergarten-teacher handwriting in red ink. This way it's easier to see what each bottle holds without having to lift out the container and search the label for the medication name.

Mom reaches to the top of the table and picks up the spreadsheet that she and Mark created two days ago so they can keep track of what pills I've taken.

"It's been eight hours since your last dose of Ativan," she says. That's for anxiety. "Do you want one now?"

"Yes," I sniff. "Can I take an Ambien, too?" I took one two hours ago, but it didn't do its job of putting me to sleep.

"Did you take one earlier?" she asks.

"No," I lie. I'm thinking that if I double up, maybe it will knock me out for a couple of hours. My body aches for sleep after being awake for nearly three days.

My mom hands over two little white pills. I slip them under my tongue and let them dissolve so the medicine will absorb more quickly into my bloodstream—a trick I learned years ago when I struggled with a serious addiction to prescription pills. The medicine creates a bitter, chalky paste in my mouth and a sinking burn in my belly. Having to take all these pills has reignited my addiction after five years of sobriety. I sip water from the small, green plastic cup that never leaves my bedside. That tiny cup has to be filled at least twenty times a day because my hands and arms are too weak to hold anything larger without dropping or spilling it. If things get any worse, I'll be demoted to a sippy cup.

My mother whispers to me for about twenty minutes to distract me from my panic. She's saying something about how I used to try to climb onto the countertops when I was a toddler and that one time she found me sitting on top of the refrigerator. I attempt to follow her line of conversation but have trouble making sense of her words. Mark holds me until my hysterics subside. Seeing me mellow out, my mom leaves our bedroom, saying she's going to try to catch up on a little sleep.

"I need to pee," I say, feeling the drugs begin to take effect.

Mark helps me out of bed and grabs my waist from behind to help me walk down the hall to the bathroom. Each step begins with a fit and start until I've taken a few and my gait levels out to a heavy Frankenstein shuffle.

Afterward, Mark helps me up and back to bed, where a miracle occurs. I fall asleep. I enjoy a drugged, dreamless rest for an unbelievable seven hours before I wake up crying in pain and fear and the cycle starts all over again.

This routine—or some slight variation on it—has been the story of our lives for four months now. I have been to the emergency room or admitted to the hospital four times in three months, since we moved in December from San Francisco to our new home in Los Angeles. Each time I go in, the ER triage nurse goes through the familiar litany of questions.

"What brings you to the emergency room?"

"I'm having an MS flare," I answer flatly.

"What are your symptoms?" the nurse will ask, and I will go through the list yet again.

"Excruciating pain in my neck, upper and mid back. My legs and arms are weak, tingling and numb. I have no sensation in my belly . . . it feels like all of my internal organs are dead. You could stab me with a sword through my midsection and I don't think I'd feel it, except on my skin, which is hypersensitive to even the gentlest touch. My balance is off and I can't walk right. I'm having cognitive problems—trouble with short-term memory and concentration. I'm so fatigued and weak I can't get out of bed most days. I have to pee at least two times an hour and occasionally have problems controlling my bowels. My vision is blurry and I'm having vertigo."

"Is this the normal pattern when your MS flares, or are you having new symptoms?" the nurse will ask, a soft look of pity in her eyes.

"This has been the norm," I say. It's been the damn norm for too long.

Each time, the treatment protocol is the same. They will hook me up to IVs, order MRIs, and shoot me full of Dilaudid (which is pharmaceutical-grade heroin) to give me a temporary break from the pain. I'm sensitive to most narcotic pain medicine, so they'll also shoot me up with Benadryl to ensure I don't scratch my skin off. They'll give me a shot of Ativan for anxiety. During one stay, they hit me with 1,000 milligrams of IV Solu-Medrol, a powerful combination of steroids, for five days straight. The steroids gave me some relief for four days, offering a glimmer of hope that things were getting better, but then I crashed. Not only did the steroids not work, but they had an agonizing side effect, hurling me into a state where I alternated between severe suicidal depression and mania.

Each time I leave the hospital with another prescription or two added to the ever-growing list of drugs I take each day—often as many as fifteen to twenty pills in a twenty-four-hour period, depending on how bad the pain is and how many panic attacks I have. I wouldn't mind taking all the pills if they helped, but my symptoms persist, and with each flare-up I feel more desperate.

Right now, my mom and Mark are very concerned about my state of mind. Not only am I depressed, I'm also having what appear to be psychotic episodes where I'm not in touch with reality. I talk high-speed nonsense, repeating myself over and over again. Mark phones the neurology resident who saw me during the last hospital visit and is given a referral to a new neurologist—a specialist in pain management, addiction, and MS. This is the fourth neurologist we've consulted since arriving in Los Angeles four months ago.

The next day, Mom, Mark, and I arrive at Dr. N's office, check in at the front desk, and sit down in the electric-blue padded chairs to wait our turn. We're surprised when the nurse calls us only a few minutes later.

Dr. N sits behind his desk and greets us with a friendly smile. He has a fine dusting of white hair combed neatly over the top of his head and wears bifocals that magnify his shiny blue eyes to three times their normal size. He is a slightly pot-bellied man, easily pushing 80. Immediately, I feel myself relax in his presence—he is clearly not rushed. Leaning forward in his chair, he begins to ask me questions: Where, precisely, is the pain? What is the nature of the pain—burning, stabbing, or aching? On a scale of one to ten, ten being the worst pain you've ever experienced, how would you rate your pain right now? Question after question after question. He takes what is by far the most detailed medical history anyone's ever taken of me, covering everything from my childhood illnesses to details of my psychiatric history.

When I tell him I'm not accustomed to a doctor spending so much time with me, he says, "I've been practicing medicine for fifty years. I refuse to turn into one of those doctors who stops listening to patients because they don't have the time." He listens patiently to my long answers, asking Mark or my mother for clarification at times, and scribbles notes like mad on a yellow legal pad. After an hour, his investigation finally complete, he puts his pen down and shakes out his right hand.

"Is there anything you'd like to tell me that you think I missed?"

"No, I don't think so," I reply, stunned. *This guy is from another time. They really don't make doctors like this anymore.* I'm used to being ushered out after a scant fifteen-minute appointment and sent home with yet another prescription.

Dr. N tells me to go into his examination room next door and put on a gown so he can take a look at me. He enters the room and proceeds to do the most thorough neurological exam of all the ones I have had. Slowly and deliberately, he performs the standard neurological tests. Then he does what he calls the "old-school swab-and-stab test," in which he touches every square inch of my skin with either a cotton ball or a blunted safety pin, asking again and again: Sharp or soft? Sharp or soft? This is his way of determining exactly where in my spinal cord the damage might be. Apparently it is the rare neurologist who investigates so painstakingly.

At last he finishes and tells me to get dressed and go back into his office with my mom and Mark so we can all talk. At this point, I have been with him for more than ninety minutes. I can't believe he is going to give me still more of his time.

Once we're all seated back in his office, Dr. N offers his observations.

"I'm very concerned about the combination of drugs you're on," he tells me, "particularly given your history of addiction." On the plus side, despite my long list of complaints, most of my nerves are intact. And, based on his initial examination, it appears my nervous system is resilient and pretty good at repairing itself. *Finally, a little good news.* Then he tells me that he's never heard an MS patient report the level of pain that I am experiencing. In fact, until recent years, pain was not even a widely accepted symptom of the disease. Dr. N asks me if any previous doctor ever mentioned that pain was unusual in MS patients. Well, no, none of them had, but I was beginning to suspect that there were a few things my previous doctors hadn't mentioned.

I begin to feel sorry for myself. It's not bad enough I have this progressive degenerative disease—which, in the worst case, will leave me paralyzed, blind, or dead and, in the best case, will likely mean managing unpredictable flare-ups of symptoms—I have to be in terrible pain, too? Figures.

Dr. N wants to contact a psychiatrist to consult on my case and calls right there on the spot to make an appointment with his colleague, Dr. S. He suggests some adjustments to dosages on my meds and tells me he will call me after my appointment with Dr. S to discuss our next steps. I follow my mother out of Dr. N's office, bracing one hand against the wall to steady myself. Dr. N watches me walk down the hall and suggests that a cane would be a wise purchase. "Your balance is clearly affected. You don't want to fall down. A cane will help you feel safer."

Mark and I argue in the car on the way home about the cane while my mother sits quietly in the backseat.

"I don't want a fucking cane," I spit at Mark. "I'm 35! I don't want to look like an old woman."

Mark pulls into a pharmacy parking lot anyway and goes in to make the purchase. He gets back in the car and hands me a hideous-looking cane with a brown, black, and gold fake-marble finish on it. "You're using it from now on and that's final. I don't want you to get hurt just because you have too much pride."

"I agree, Cami," says my mom quietly. "It's not worth risking falling down and hurting yourself. Just use the cane."

"You could have at least gotten a plain black one. This thing is ugly as hell," I whine as I toss the cane against the car door and fold my arms across my chest.

"That's the only one they had. Who cares what it looks like as long as it will keep you safe?"

"I care," I say through a fresh burst of tears. "I care what it looks like." Then I proceed to cry all the way home.

I see Dr. S the very next day (ugly new cane in tow), and he turns out to be just as thorough as Dr. N. My mom and I sit on his black leather sofa and listen as he gives us his opinion in his thoughtful, measured speech. He thinks I should go into the hospital again—this time for an eight-day medical detox, to get me off most of the drugs so we can start over with a clean slate. Getting off the meds could yield a crucial bit of information, namely, whether my pain is a result of nervous system damage or whether it's a by-product of the combination of drugs I'm taking. Whether or not my pain subsides when I detox will give us our answer.

The truth is, I really don't know *how* I feel anymore, I'm so doped up most of the time. After seeing these two new doctors, I have the sense that I can trust them, though, so I agree to the hospital stay. I'll be admitted through the psychiatric ward at UCLA Medical Center the next day. Both Dr. S and Dr. N warn me that things will likely get worse before they get better—the detox will be painful and intense. I'm not overjoyed by this news, but I know this is the right step. I keep imagining how good it will feel to be free of all those prescription bottles.

That night, I call my friend and spiritual mentor Mbali Creazzo. Mbali would call herself a "medicine woman." She is South African, but her family moved to England when she was three because of apartheid. She has a "wise woman" way about her: quiet, peaceful, insightful. She chooses her words carefully. She may not seem all that remarkable when you're in her presence, but she has a ripple effect on you. She is the person who introduced me to the concept of the 29 Gifts "prescription," and in many ways I feel I owe her my life.

Mark and I met Mbali in 2005, when we knew her as just Toni, our next-door neighbor. We were living near Lake Merritt in Oakland, to get a break from the frenetic bustle of San Francisco. A couple of times a week she and I would carpool for the twenty-minute trip to work. I had a high-stress job with an ad agency, and she worked at The Institute for Health and Healing at California Pacific Hospital. She is actually one of the innovative healers who helped guide and shape the programs at the institute, where they marry Western medicine with various forms of alternative medicine. We were friendly, but not really friends. About six months after we met, she made plans to go to South Africa for a couple of weeks to visit some relatives. She knocked on our door and politely asked whether Mark and I would feed her cats while she was away. We were glad to help.

The first time I walked into Toni's apartment, I nearly stumbled over a large altar on the floor by the front door. Beside a vase of flowers stood an open bottle of vodka, which perplexed me because I knew she didn't drink. There were also a bowl full of ash, piles of rocks and shells, and a number of African statues that looked fierce and intimidating.

I had been exploring various forms of spirituality over the years and have several friends with altars in their homes, but most of them just held some pretty crystals and maybe some angel cards or even a cross. But the contents of this altar freaked me out a little. I knew there was nothing to be afraid of; Toni was a caring, loving woman who lived to help people. Regardless, while I tended to the cats, I skirted around that altar, giving it a wide berth. I wanted to ask her about it when she got back but decided against it. I figured if she wanted to tell me about her spiritual practice, she would.

When Toni got home from South Africa, she announced that she would now go by the name "Mbali," pronounced *em-BALL-ee*. Over the years, I had several friends who traveled to India to meet gurus and came back using new names. Another friend changed her name just because she didn't like the one her parents gave her. So we started calling Toni "Mbali" and didn't think much of it. She looked the same, but something on that trip had apparently changed her. How much so, I would find out later.

A few months later, Mbali returned the favor and fed our cats when Mark and I went to Mexico for our wedding and honeymoon. I had been working like a fiend. At my extremely demanding job as creative strategy director of an advertising agency, I made a lot of money, but the pressure was constant and the hours were long—sixty hours would be a short week for me. In the month before the wedding, while I was finishing a big new pitch, I kept noticing that my mind didn't seem to be working right. The words were in my head, but sometimes I couldn't get them out. My hands hurt and were very stiff. I would will my fingers to move over the keyboard, but they wouldn't hit the right keys. Chalking it up to stress, I managed to wind up the intense work weeks and get on the plane to Mexico. Mark and I enjoyed three amazing, relaxing weeks in Playa del Carmen, celebrating with forty of our family members and friends.

Then we flew home and our life disintegrated in a matter of weeks.

I may only have noticed those weird symptoms for a few weeks in 2006, but looking back it's now obvious to me that I had been having flare-ups of MS symptoms over the previous fifteen years. Sometimes my toes or fingers would go numb. Or my whole body would feel the way your foot does when it falls asleep. I'd have vomiting spells that were so bad I'd lose 20 pounds in a week. I'd be so tired that I'd need to stop three times to rest during the two-block walk to the bus stop. The doctors always told me there was nothing physiologically wrong, that it was just stress. The main prescription they gave me was to relax.

So in 1997, when I was 24, a year after moving to San Francisco from Nebraska, I began to seek alternative treatments. During the decade I lived in the Bay Area before my diagnosis, I regularly saw an acupuncturist, several different massage therapists, a chiropractor, a hypnotherapist, a meditation teacher, and a nutrition counselor, plus I practiced yoga at least five days a week, all of which had tremendous therapeutic benefit. I firmly believe that if it weren't for this team of holistic practitioners, I would be much worse off today. I think their help kept the MS at bay, but only for so long. It was no match for the overdriven lifestyle I lived. There is a strong connection between high levels of stress over extended periods of time and autoimmune diseases. Scientists are still studying this connection, but I believe that if I had made different lifestyle choices, it is possible I may not have developed full-blown MS.

While Mark and I were on our honeymoon, I developed a urinary tract infection. We had four days left in Mexico, and I wanted to wait till we were back in the States to treat it. By that time it was pretty bad. (I've since learned that a UTI is a common trigger for an MS flare.) The infection cleared up after I saw a doctor, but three days later I woke up and my hands simply didn't work. I couldn't bend them; they were stuck like claws. Over the next couple of days I felt tremendous fatigue. I could hardly get anything done at work. By the time I lost the vision in my right eye, I found myself back in the hands of mainstream doctors after a pretty long absence.

My diagnosis of MS came just one month after my wedding day. Three neurologists in white coats took turns looking into my right eye and commenting on the degradation they could see on my optic nerve. They took me through a few standard neurological tests. Tap your index finger and thumb together. Walk heel to toe. Touch your nose with your index finger. One of the top neurologists at the UCSF Medical Center confirmed the diagnosis for me by showing me pictures of my brain from the MRI scans they took.

"You see this hook-shaped white lesion here?" he asked, pointing to his computer screen. "That's a classic MS lesion. Judging from your history of symptoms, I'd estimate you've had MS for more than a decade."

"A decade!" exclaimed Mark, stunned. "Shouldn't someone have caught this sooner?"

"I don't think she's ever had enough symptoms present at one time to lead to an accurate diagnosis," replied the doctor. So there really wasn't anyone to blame, but that didn't stop me from being angry at all the doctors I saw over the years who told me I was suffering from nothing more than stress.

Now here I sit on the phone with Mbali. It is the night before my psych ward stay to detox, and she listens intently and lets me cry for a while. Then, in her British lilt, she attempts to pull me out of my self-pity.

"Cami, I think you need to stop thinking about yourself."

For a few seconds, I'm shocked silent. I imagine Mbali on the other end of the phone, sitting near her unique altar, her silver hair and bronze skin reflecting in the soft light of her apartment. She's probably wearing one of the beautiful, colorful necklaces she makes and smiling at my stunned reaction.

"Thinking about myself?" I howl. I start in on her about what a wreck I am, what a wreck my body is, telling her I don't have room to think about anything except myself right now.

"I know, that's the problem," she says. "If you spend all of your time and energy focusing on your pain, you're feeding the disease. You're making it worse by putting all of your attention there."

I absorb this information quietly.

"Cami," she says, her voice soft and soothing but her words hitting me hard, "you are falling deeper and deeper into a black hole. I'm going to give you a tool to help you dig yourself out."

"What should I do?" I ask.

"I have a prescription for you. I want you to give away 29 gifts in 29 days."

I blink and consider this for a moment before deciding it is stupid. For one thing, I'm going into the hospital for eight days—how can I give anything away there?

"There will be others at the hospital with you," Mbali counters. "You can give to them. These gifts don't have to be material things."

I continue to insist that I need to focus all my energy on my own healing, while Mbali calmly points out what I'm forgetting: "Healing doesn't happen in a vacuum, Cami, but through our interactions with other people. By giving, you are focusing on what you have to offer others, inviting more abundance into your life. Giving of any kind is taking a positive action that begins the process of change. It will shift your energy for life."

I'm starting to tune out, wallowing in thoughts of what I am about to endure. *I'm in pain and I can't freaking walk! Are you telling me that giving away spare change or doing someone a favor will make me better? Come on!*

Mbali tells me about the effects the "challenge" of giving 29 gifts had on her when she first did it. It makes sense in a way, but I'm not really taking it in. She's saying how giving can make you humble, keep your heart open, revitalize you, that kind of thing.

In addition to giving the gifts, you're supposed to keep a journal for those 29 days. If you skip a day for some reason, she's saying it's best to start over, to release the energy that is building and allow it to begin building again.

Now, I've been into alternative medicine and spirituality for a long time, but even I have no patience for all this. And I'm in the midst of a medical crisis. Without any intention of following through, I grab my journal and write a note: "Give away 29 gifts in 29 days." I close the journal and politely say goodnight to Mbali.

The following afternoon my mother and Mark take me to the psych ward at UCLA. After I check in, there's nothing more they can do for me. My mom tells me she'll be praying for me every day, and Mark assures me he'll be back tomorrow during visiting hours after delivering my mother to the airport for her flight home to Nebraska. They leave me in a putty-colored plastic chair near the nurses' station, crying.

The eight days in the hospital are hell. I'm in a room sandwiched between a woman who is puking constantly because she's detoxing off heroin and a paranoid schizophrenic who thinks everyone who comes within 50 feet of her is trying to kill her. The idea is to taper me off my medications under a careful eye. By day three, I'm so weak that I have to get around in a wheelchair.

But I do manage to take part in all the therapy and chemical-dependency groups and even decoupage my cane during an occupational therapy session. I turn it into a bright, colorful accessory that feels like an extension of me, rather than an ugly extra appendage that I need because my legs don't work right. As planned, I go off all my medications except for Copaxone, an immunosuppressant I inject myself with daily to slow the progression of the disease. Dr. N and Dr. S decide to start me on Cymbalta, an antidepressant that also treats anxiety and neuropathic pain. Even though I am now off all the muscle relaxants, painkillers, and sedatives that can be addictive and that may have been a bad mix, I'm still in searing pain. So they were most likely not to blame. The latest set of MRI scans reveal a lesion in my thoracic spine that is probably the culprit.

By day eight, I've come to appreciate and respect my

fellow loony-bin mates. We're all trying to slay different personal demons. I have made friends with Katie, my heroin addict neighbor. Before I leave the hospital, I give her a book I brought with me called *Come Home,* a mother and daughter's story of their journey through hell and back as the daughter struggles with heroin addiction. *Always remember,* I write inside the book, *that you have your own angels looking out for you. You deserve a good life. Please make that choice for yourself.* Then I say that I hope to bump into her at an addiction support meeting sometime soon and leave her my phone number.

I hobble out of the lock-down unit into the blinding sunlight for the first time in more than a week with my fancy new cane, and I realize how lucky I am. My mind still works, even if I'm a bit impaired. I'm cheered when I look down and see my two favorite phrases, which I've affixed to the cane:

Not every adventure takes place in a storybook.

and . . .

*Actually, good things come to those who **can't** wait.*

For the first time in many, many months, I feel a little bit hopeful that I may be on the road to recovery.

When I get home, I am exhausted since I didn't sleep more than two hours a night during my detox. Despite my delirious state, Mark and I talk for hours and then make love for the first time in more than six months.

Unfortunately, the insomnia doesn't let up at home, and I continue to have problems with chronic pain, weakness, and many other symptoms. After a week, I'm still having difficulty walking. My balance is off. My legs feel wobbly and weak, allowing me to take only halting, heavy steps. When the fatigue comes on very badly, I can't even hold myself up. Once again I fall into a familiar trough of panic and despair. *Did I go through that nightmare week for nothing?! I'm 35 years old, and my body is betraying me. I should be enjoying my wonderful new husband, but I'm a wreck. It's so unfair!* Time for a first-class pity party.

One sleepless night, as I'm sitting on the couch, I decide to write in my journal. I open the lavender-flowered book and land on the page with a note I scribbled in green ink a month ago:

Give away 29 gifts in 29 days.

Oh yeah, I think, *Mbali's advice.* I look up from the notebook and this time I think, *Well, why not? Compared to what I've already been through, how hard can it be?*

I decide to go ahead and take this uncommon prescription from Mbali. I don't expect it to change things dramatically, but I doubt it will hurt me. *Who knows? Maybe it will help,* I think as I shut my journal and begin to ponder what my first gift should be.

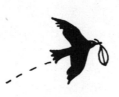

I

The Gifts

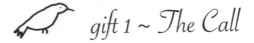

gift 1 ~ The Call

Aside from my physical symptoms, I'm starting to see how much MS has made my self-esteem plummet. I feel that I'm no longer capable of living a productive life, that I have nothing to contribute to the world. My job is gone, and with it a huge piece of my identity. Defeat seeps through me. I don't enjoy spending time with myself, so why would anyone else? I stopped reaching out to friends long ago, feeling I had nothing positive to talk about.

But I haven't changed my mind about the 29 Gifts prescription. I want to give my first gift today. *What am I going to give?* I try to recall some of what Mbali described that day when I wasn't very receptive. I walk into the kitchen to make a cup of tea when it comes to me.

I will call my friend Lauri, who also struggles with multiple sclerosis. She's an inspiration to me. Her MS has advanced more than mine. Though she's only about ten years older than I am, she's been dealing with MS since the 1970s. She has more trouble walking than I do and usually needs a walker, crutches, or her motorized scooter to get around. Yet, despite these obstacles, Lauri still gets her butt out of the house and to the gym every day at 7 a.m.

"Cami!" Lauri exclaims when she answers the phone. "It's so good to hear from you!" We end up talking for an hour, and it feels great to reconnect. As it turns out, her husband is out of town and she's feeling lonely, so I offer to visit later in the week. When I hang up the phone, I'm somehow calmer, lighter. There's even a smile on my face.

I'm still smiling when the phone rings. To my surprise, it's someone from a large philanthropy firm offering me a marketing consultant gig. These days, when I'm feeling capable, I supplement the disability insurance payments I receive each month by providing marketing assistance to start-up companies and nonprofits. I haven't had the energy to work for months, though, much less make an effort to find any clients, so this call is unexpected to say the least. "Yes, I'm definitely interested," I chirp into the mouthpiece. We begin to work out the details and make a plan to talk again in a few days.

Ha! That didn't take long. I'm tempted to link the new-found work to the call I just made to Lauri as my first gift, but I'm skeptical. It might take more than a moment for the energy in the universe to shift, after all. Nonetheless, I'm feeling pretty good and definitely up for the consulting work. I'd like to take myself out to breakfast to celebrate and to get out of the house for awhile, but I need Mark's help getting safely out of our second-floor apartment. It's filled with great Craftsman character—lots of built-in cabinetry, doors with beautiful leaded glass, woodwork stained a rich, deep hue— but it also has a dark, steep set of fourteen steps leading down to the building's front door. That's scary when your brain and limbs aren't always in sync.

Mark helps me downstairs, then drives me to a nearby café and assists me to get inside. He heads to a voiceover audition—he makes his living as a voice actor for television, films, radio, and video games. He'll pick me up in two or three hours.

There are small tables close together near the entrance, more accessible for me and my cane than the more spacious ones toward the back. "Is it okay if I sit here?" I ask the friendly-looking man wearing a blue AT&T shirt seated next to the table I'd like to claim.

"Sure, no problem."

It's my first time here. I glance at the menu. "Is there anything good here?"

"I come here all the time," he tells me, "and everything I've tried has been good." Then, eyeing my cane, he asks, "What happened? Did you have an accident?"

"No," I explain, thinking for a second how I will respond to these kinds of questions. "I have an illness. I've had a hard time walking since I moved to L.A." It's not like me to strike up a conversation with a stranger, no less to bring even more attention to my problems walking around. We make small talk while we eat our greasy diner food. He finishes before me and says goodbye as he stands to leave. I bid him farewell and dig into my hash browns.

Soon after, my waiter comes over and tells me that the AT&T man paid my bill.

Really? This kind of thing never happens to me.

"How nice," I tell the waiter. I had never even exchanged names with the guy. "Maybe people in L.A. are nicer than they get credit for."

The waiter laughs as he clears my table and I dig through my purse to find a tip for him, finally coming up with $3.00

in change. I had intended to pay my tab with my credit card and write his tip onto the receipt.

Watching the other diners while I sip my orange juice, it suddenly occurs to me that I have a couple of hours to kill before Mark can pick me up. I can't believe I forgot to bring a book or my journal. It's a quick fall from freebie to frustration, but I don't want to lose the positive vibe of this uplifting morning. *Okay, Cami, you're not going to sit here doing nothing,* I tell myself. No, I'm not. I'm going to try walking home with my cane.

As is true most days, I'm in pain today and my legs are very stiff. Nothing different there. What's different is that I consider the options, and sitting at a tiny table in this diner with nothing to do for two hours loses out to trying to walk home on my own. I have my cell phone with me, and can always tell Mark to pick me up from a bench or someone's front yard along the way if I have to stop.

Just focus on taking one step at a time, I think, and set out across the parking lot. I cross Santa Monica Boulevard and don't quite make it across before the WALK sign changes to DON'T WALK—not soon enough to put me in any danger, but enough to warn me that I could get stuck at a bad spot. I keep going, step by step. It takes me forty-five minutes, but to my amazement I make the whole six blocks and arrive triumphantly at our building. I haul myself up those steep stairs on all fours and sit down on the top step, resting my head on my cane. A sob of relief escapes me. *I just walked home alone! I didn't really think I could, but I did. What else might I be capable of?*

I feel tired and emotional, but when Mark gets home I gush all about my morning and we both feel happy.

"That's fantastic, Cami! I'm so proud of you!" he beams.

Somehow we get through the whole afternoon without any disagreements, which is unusual these days. There's often a lot of arguing in our house because we're both so frustrated with my physical state. I barely remember the last peaceful day we spent together.

That evening, I attend an addiction support meeting. My long history of substance abuse started when I was all of 12 years old and got drunk for the first time. I was always looking for a way not to feel what I was feeling. I tried to be an alcoholic, but I wasn't a good drinker. It always made me puke, or I'd black out. I progressed to marijuana, a *lot* of marijuana, and then I got addicted to prescription medication like sleeping pills, anti-anxiety drugs, and pain medications. I cleaned up from time to time—once for a period of two years and another time for five years. But during the twelve years that I have been trying to live sober, I've had more relapses than I can count.

I started my sobriety date over after leaving the hospital and getting off the latest set of drugs. I'd definitely taken more of them than my doctors had prescribed. I like to attend meetings when I can get myself out of the house. Mark had substance abuse issues in the past, too, and in fact we met through an addiction support group. For him, sobriety seems to come more easily, though: He stopped seven years ago and never picked up a drink or drug again.

At tonight's meeting, a woman named Ingrid stands up and tells the story of how she healed her relationship with her abusive, alcoholic mother. Just two weeks ago Ingrid had returned from attending her mother's funeral in England. She reveals that her mother died from complications related to multiple sclerosis.

Ingrid has the rapt attention of the small crowd as she speaks in her cockney accent: "Me Mum suffered greatly the last ten years of her life. She had very little company except for the people who were paid to take care of her. I arrived at the hospital when she was very close to death. Tears came to Mum's eyes, like she was waiting for me to get there so she could let go." Tears came to my eyes, too, as I listened to this moving story told in a no-nonsense style. She had grown up with a mother who had physically abused her, but Ingrid found the freedom that comes with forgiveness and had managed to build a relationship with her mother in sobriety. Ingrid had been sober for more than a dozen years.

I chat with her and a few other people after the meeting, collecting phone numbers. I'm a little rusty at this—it's the first time I've made any concentrated effort to make friends since arriving in Los Angeles four months ago.

After I return I'm still feeling up to going out to dinner with Mark. Later, lying in bed next to him, I reflect quietly on what turned out to be a pretty amazing day. *I was out of the house three times today; that's so much better than once every three or four days like usual. I called Lauri, my first of the 29 Gifts. I walked all the way home from the diner. I may even have made a couple of new friends at the support group meeting. Mark takes such good care of me . . . he really tries hard.*

I turn over contentedly, and for the first time in weeks, I sleep through the night, soundly, undrugged—a full eight hours—and wake up actually glad to greet the day. I don't know whether it has anything to do with Gift 1, but I'm already thinking about the possibilities for Gift 2.

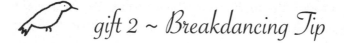

gift 2 ~ Breakdancing Tip

Everything I do these days takes twice as long as it should. I remember when I could just grab a bottle of shampoo and squeeze some out, for instance. Now I leave the bottle open because I don't have the strength in my hand to flip the lid up, and this morning I've already dropped it twice. It's almost as much of a balancing act as getting the water temperature right—I miss luxurious hot showers, but heat triggers my symptoms, so I keep the water as cool as I can stand. I'm getting ready for my appointment with Dr. Kim, my acupuncturist, and I'm running behind.

My limbs respond sluggishly. At this point, my main problems are extreme fatigue, problems with balance, problems moving my legs and hands, and cognitive challenges, meaning I can't concentrate well and have a poor memory. I often begin an activity and forget what I'm doing before the task is complete. I'll sit down to my computer surprised to see an unsent e-mail I began hours earlier. Or I'll leave things on the stove to burn because I forget I'm cooking something. Mark often gets frustrated because he has to remind me of conversations we've had that I can't recall.

I'm sitting on the bathtub floor and lathering up with Dr. Bronner's peppermint soap when the front door buzzes and I realize that Dr. Kim is on time but I'm not. She's been picking me up for my appointments because she just moved her office, and her new place isn't as close to me as her old one was. As if that weren't generous enough, she has not been charging me for the daily sessions I've had with her since leaving the hospital. I feel bad, but I just can't pay her right now. She keeps insisting that she's treating me now, when I need it, and that when I'm feeling better and can work again, I can pay.

I finish rinsing, turn off the water and carefully work my way out of the tub to dry off and dress. Grabbing my cane, I make my way down the steps and out the front door, where Dr. Kim is sitting on my stoop, waiting patiently.

"I'm sorry. I'm running late," I say as I lock the door.

"Is okay," she says. She stands up to take my free arm and helps me to her car.

Dr. Kim is Korean, and though she's been practicing acupuncture in Los Angeles for seven years, her English is a bit spotty. She understands me relatively well, but sometimes has a hard time making herself understood. We often communicate through hand signals and acting things out, as if we're playing charades.

"Thank you so much for the ride," I say once we're moving east down Sunset Boulevard.

"Is okay," she says again. "How you feel today?"

"Stronger," I reply. Automatically, I list the answers to the questions she asks me every day: "Appetite good. Sleep last night good. Energy and balance a little better."

"Good. Good. Is good," Dr. Kim says as she slows to a stop at a red light. She turns her head toward me, her blunt black bob swinging from side to side. She has a very girlish face, even though at 37, she's two years older than I am. "And poo-poo . . . you go poo-poo?"

"Once last night. Once this morning," I say, and she breaks into a huge smile of victory.

"Oh, is very, very good!" She bounces excitedly in her seat and then settles down when the traffic light turns green.

Dr. Kim is obsessed with my bowel movements, or more accurately, my lack of them. Sometimes I go four to six days without one. She is on a mission to get me pooping regularly with her bitter-tasting herbal concoctions. Apparently, it's beginning to work.

When we pull up at her new office, I feel renewed guilt that Dr. Kim has driven in busy L.A. traffic from her new office in Koreatown all the way to Hollywood to get me. And she will have to make the trip again to take me home. Asking for help makes me uneasy, but I haven't driven since early November, when I crashed a friend's car into a cement wall because my right foot didn't move off the gas pedal when my brain told it to.

"Dr. Kim, I'm sorry you have to do all this extra driving for me," I apologize as we enter her office.

She helps me settle into a chair and then sits down behind her desk. On a previous visit I'd brought her a cute succulent plant from my windowsill as an office-warming present, and it's sitting on a shelf behind her, my handmade "Thank You" note in orange marker is still propped up in the dirt with a toothpick.

"Cami, no worry," she says. "You not just patient. You my first American friend. I helping you. This driving, treatment, is gift. You accept. Make me happy."

I am quiet for a moment and my eyes well up without warning. I am so touched by her generosity, and I'm starting to understand that I may need to accept help from others a lot. Just as I am trying to give consciously now, I will try to receive consciously, too.

"Thank you," I say through my tears. "Thank you so much."

"Is okay," she says and hands me a tissue. "Now treatment. You get undressed. On table. I wash my hands. Be back."

I climb onto Dr. Kim's table and feel my body relax as she begins to massage my feet and back. She inserts about fifteen thin little needles all over my back and into my heels. I feel a zing of energy as each needle pokes through my skin and an occasional flash of pain. The treatment lasts about an hour, and I accept the ride back home with no further apologies for needing it . . . just words of gratitude. This is an art, this learning to receive help graciously.

When I get home I eat lunch and then take a nap. The phone wakes me up.

It's my friend Elline, who has also recently moved to L.A. from the Bay Area. We have not managed to meet up since she arrived because I've been so sick. She offers to come over so we can go for a short walk. Yes! It's very important for me to walk whenever I have the energy so I can continue to rehabilitate myself and maintain the physical function I have left. Walking requires coordination of nerves, muscles, and tendons all firing at once, and the more I practice keeping these vital functions in synch, the better my chances of staying out of a wheelchair over the long haul.

As we step outside at 4 p.m., it is still warm, but fortunately the blazing L.A. sun isn't straight overhead anymore. After we walk a few blocks, my gait feels smoother and I manage to keep up with Elline, my cane tapping the ground with each step. It's so nice to have someone to walk with—and it relieves me from worrying that I won't be able to make it back. We follow the pink stars down Hollywood Boulevard until we reach the Kodak Theater, where they televise the Oscars. We see a crowd of people gathering on the sidewalk, some of them tapping their feet to a lively hip-hop beat. They are all watching a group of nine young men line up for a street performance.

We stop to watch their show, an awesome display of breakdancing prowess. The guys bounce off the cement like SuperBalls and bring so much energy to their performance that the large crowd begins to cheer and dance along with them. One kid goes into a backbend, then kicks up, balancing on one hand, then the other. The dancers stop the music after three enthusiastic numbers and announce that it's *almost* time for the grand finale, but first they'd like to collect donations. The leader of the troupe, a beautiful Latino boy of about 18, begins to work the crowd like an auctioneer. I am surprised that I feel moved to reach for the emergency $5 bill tucked in the waistband of my drawstring pants. I don't normally hand out money on the street. The young man with the purple velvet money bag walks directly up to me as if he can read my mind. I pluck the money from its hiding place and hand him the five. He winks, making me blush, then shakes my hand and turns to face the crowd. Waving the $5 bill around madly for all to see, he points back at me and yells, "Hey, this rich white lady just gave me five bucks!"

This sets the tone and other people start whipping out $5 bills. Many in the crowd are matching, even bettering, my donation. The breakdancing finale involves two teenage girls and one boy of about 8, plucked from the spectators to join the show. The crowd loves it.

I decide to call Mbali when I get home, to let her know that I've taken her suggestion and to go over the ground rules again. "You know," I tell her, "I never had any intention of doing the 29 gifts, but I started yesterday and good things are happening already!"

I can hear the smile in her voice. "I'm not surprised, Cami," she says. "No matter how much we have materially, we are often in a place of scarcity: we never think we have enough or that we're good enough. Instead of getting lost in a sense of *lack,* once we realize we are part of something bigger, it becomes clear we have many gifts to offer the world."

This time I feel truly connected to what Mbali is telling me. "Twenty-nine gifts in twenty-nine days. Are you writing your gifts down?" she asks.

She explained that it's a good idea to keep a journal to record the experience and to be *mindful* of both the journal and the gifts so that they can do their work of transforming you. She mentioned, too, that starting each day with a short meditation and an affirmation can help. It has been a while since I have meditated, but I looked forward to getting back to it. As for affirmations, something as simple as "Today I give with joy" or "Today I give with patience" can set the right tone.

The gifts can be anything from spare change to a kind word or thought. Along with giving them, the prescription involves thinking of things to be grateful for each day and reflecting on the tradition of giving in your family.

"Gratitude keeps your heart open. When you give with an open heart, you receive the profound gift of humility," Mbali explains.

I'm part of something now, and I'm ready to get swept up in its momentum.

gift 3 ~ More than One Way to Dance

Mark and I sit in the car outside a cute little ranch-style home with a long black metal ramp leading to the front door. My belly seizes up in fear. *This can't happen to me. I don't want to depend on ramps, walkers, and wheelchairs.*

I am here to visit Lauri, the friend I called on the first day of my giving challenge. She's an MS sufferer, too, or maybe I should say an MS *thriver.* She continues to pursue life with gusto despite the physical limitations she faces. There are two kinds of "patients" I've met during the long struggle with both my physical and mental health. Some allow their diagnosis to define them, falling victim to their disease and living at the mercy of what the doctors tell them. Then there are those who face their illness head-on, taking responsibility for their own healing and choosing to live a thriving life. I myself have fallen into one or the other camp at different times and have certainly spent the last six months in the victim club. *God, am I ready to get rid of that.*

That's in part why I'm here today. I've learned through mental health recovery programs that one of the best ways to change is to surround yourself with people who live as you aspire to. Lauri has guts and a drive for life that I desperately want to rekindle for myself.

It's 11:20 a.m., much later than I planned on arriving. I've never been an on-the-dot person anyway, but MS makes timeliness more difficult. Lauri is all too familiar with the daily challenges I face and isn't upset when I call to let her know I'm running behind.

Lauri and I met in an MS Society workshop called the Optimal Living Program and hit it off instantly. But this is my first visit to her house and the first time I've confronted a ramp leading to a friend's front door. Mark helps me up the ramp and I am nearly knocked to the floor by Chip, her Australian Shepherd, who is clearly excited to have visitors. Inside, a heap of tween-sized clothing, evidence of Lauri's 12-year-old daughter, covers the top of the grand piano in a far corner of the room, an open space that serves as living room, sunroom, and dining room. I plop down next to Lauri on her pretty floral couch while Mark sets down my tote bag, which is bulging with all the items I intend to give her today, things I collected around my house before we left: organic strawberries, a book, some of Dr. Kim's magic poop pills. Mark makes sure we're situated before heading off. He looks relieved to know I will be in someone's care for the day.

"I love your house," I tell Lauri. "It's adorable."

"Thanks," she replies flatly.

"What's up?" I ask. "Are you having a bad day?"

Lauri's energy seems low. Her long, curly brown hair is a bit plastered down, as if she didn't take time to primp. She is wearing no makeup. Even her clothes are muted—a light blue tank top and white cotton pants. Usually she is decked out in bright-colored prints. It strikes me how thin Lauri is when I see her in these unfamiliar clothes.

"I'm having a bad day in my head," she says. "Sometimes I just feel like my days slide by . . . pointlessly. I miss working. I miss that feeling of accomplishment."

I'm so surprised that someone like Lauri would feel this way. "But you *are* accomplished," I tell her. "You sing in your choir. You're a great mom. For heaven's sake, you work out at the gym *every day!* You're accomplishing more than many able-bodied people out there."

"I just wish there was something I could do for work. I want to feel productive again," she says, leaning back against the sofa. "You know, I used to be a professional dancer and massage therapist, but MS robbed me of my career. You can't dance in a wheelchair."

I've heard her talk about this feeling in our workshops. I feel something click into place as I listen to her story one more time, and I interrupt her in the middle of it.

"Lauri—are you open to some feedback?" I ask. This is a technique I learned from the many therapists I've seen over the years, getting permission from someone before offering advice. Lauri nods her head.

"I think you need to stop telling this story. A wise mentor once told me to be mindful of the stories I tell over and over because they are indicative of the thought patterns and beliefs that limit me. I don't think your MS robbed you of your ability to dance," I say to her. "You *chose* to stop dancing because you couldn't dance as well as you wanted. You could still dance in your wheelchair, maybe not professionally, but you *could* dance. You just *choose not to* because the dancing doesn't look the way it used to."

Lauri is quiet. Watching her, I'm worried that maybe I've pushed too far. *Who am I to preach what to do?*

Only one of Lauri's big brown eyes is focused straight at me because the MS makes it hard for her to control her eye movements. At first her inability to hold eye contact made me uncomfortable. My snap judgment was that she might have cognitive issues and find it hard to follow a conversation. But Lauri's mind is sharp, and she has helped me learn that physical symptoms often bear no relation to a person's abilities.

"I miss dancing so much," she says.

"What if you choreographed some movement and dance sequences for people who have limited mobility and taught classes?" I ask.

Lauri looks intrigued by this idea. We brainstorm for a while about how she might start to do something like this. I tell her about a dance class for differently-abled children that I once observed. The kids were amazing. The ones with mental limitations were able to help those with physical limitations. Those on crutches helped those in wheelchairs. I attended the class several times as an observer and took photographs for an article I was working on for my college newspaper. During the weeks I was there, the kids were learning a routine choreographed to John Lennon's "Imagine," and they were preparing for a public performance.

"You know, Cami, maybe I could start a class," Lauri says slowly. "I might be able to get some help through my church . . ."

"Yeah! Exactly. Why don't you make some calls to local dance studios and do some research online to see if anything similar exists already?" I recommend. I have fallen right into my role as business coach and start-up consultant. I particularly like helping women launch new businesses. Now that I'm giving Lauri suggestions for taking action, I realize how much I miss working. I'm suddenly cheered when I remember the surprise call from the philanthropic organization.

"Have you had other ideas about what you might do for work?"

"Well, I know how to adapt and keep living an active life with a disability," she says. "I've thought about doing some counseling or coaching to help aging baby boomers maintain active lives."

"That's a great idea!" I exclaim. "The dance classes could be just one of the programs you offer to people." We brainstorm some more in that direction.

Soon, Lauri is smiling and bursting with ideas for herself. She only needed to scratch the surface for all these thoughts to come tumbling out. As I listen to her ambitions, I realize that I've just given my gift for the day. I showed up with a bag full of stuff to give my friend, but the real gift is the notion of possibility offered to someone who needs a little boost. I pull the items out of the bag that I brought and give them to Lauri, then start folding some of her daughter's clothes and putting a few things away. I'm getting a little tired, though, so I offer to come back another day to help her clean out and organize her closet.

"I haven't thrown out any clothing since the 1980s! I desperately need to purge," she explains. "I've kept everything I used to wear before my MS progressed, back when life was good . . ."

I know what she means about hanging on to the things from "before." Life was good for me before MS, and the truth is, I took it for granted. I had a huge community of friends in San Francisco, a strong yoga practice, spiritual mentors who meant a lot to me. I was always taking classes or practicing meditation, and I knew a lot of people from that world. My job was exciting and challenging—I never had the same day twice. I loved throwing big dinner parties. Those days are gone, but this time I resist the usual plunge into negativity.

"Lauri, our lives are good now. We're just not appreciating the good things. I know I spend too much time looking at what's wrong instead of what's right," I confess.

She agrees that this is true, and we vow to help each other shift our thinking from dwelling on the negatives to focusing on the positives.

gift 4 ~ Compassion and Cake

The good mood doesn't last long.

With Mark off at an audition, I'm alone in our apartment with my pain and depression. I don't feel content, happy, or generous—just run down from my all-day visit with Lauri yesterday. I am still learning how to conserve my energy, which is a big topic of discussion in the Optimal Living Program workshops I've been taking with Lauri. The occupational therapists have been teaching us that it's important to pace ourselves. Familiar resentment burns a hole in my belly. *I'm so fucking irritated. Why do I have to be tired? Why can't my body just let me do what I want to, when I want to do it?* I catch myself as I complete that thought. What did I promise Lauri just yesterday? That I will do my best to focus on what's right instead of what's wrong in my life. *Remember, life is good. All is well.* I decide to allow myself to stay in today to rest and recharge.

The only thing I have scheduled is dinner with Ingrid, the woman I met at the addiction support group two days ago. *If I'm still feeling tired at 3 p.m.,* I tell myself, *it's okay to cancel.* Then I close my eyes and sleep until 1:00 p.m., when I finally get up, only because I have to pee. I go to the bathroom and then make a smoothie, which is all I feel capable of "cooking." After I drink it I lie down on the couch, alone with my thoughts, which go south quickly.

This week I'm forcing myself to find things to be grateful for when my thoughts start to spiral downward. On some days it's a stretch to find anything. Today I pull my journal off the nearby shelf, grab a pen, and start to make a list. It's hard to think of anything other than what's in front of my eyes, so why not start with that?

1. I have a lovely two-bedroom apartment.
2. Somehow, I live in the one apartment in L.A. that doesn't have floor-to-ceiling mirrored sliding doors on all the closets, which I hate.
3. Everybody who's owned this place has kept the luscious period details intact.
4. I have two cuddly cats who are thrilled to lie around with me and let me pet them.

I put my pen down to rub Habib's little white kitty belly as she stretches out alongside me. I think of one more thing to add, a biggie:

5. My husband washes all the dishes, takes out the garbage, and does all the laundry without ever complaining about my lack of wifely abilities in those areas.

Still exhausted but a little more upbeat, I reach for the phone and call Ingrid to cancel our dinner. When she answers, I can hear in her voice that she is upset.

Instead of launching in with my own sob story, I ask, "Ingrid, are you crying?"

It's awkward asking. I really don't know this woman. Yes, I heard her moving story about making peace with her mom, but we've never *talked*. That's the thing about recovery meetings. You hear each other bare your soul to the group, but you don't often share the day-to-day details that weave true friendships.

"I've been missing me mum a lot today," Ingrid says.

She's worried that her mom is still in pain on the "other side." I listen to Ingrid's story of her mother's painful life. Afflicted with MS, she was bed-bound for her last ten years. Other than the visits from Ingrid, when she could make it back to England, her mom only had the company of nurses and aides. She couldn't bathe, feed herself, or even go to the bathroom alone. After numerous lung infections over the years, she eventually succumbed to pneumonia in her mid-sixties. Being stuck in bed made it hard for her body to fight the infection and clear out her lungs.

Whenever I hear a story of someone with MS that has progressed to that level, I get scared. I know that many people with MS stay functional their entire lives. Some go years at a time without any major flare-ups of symptoms. So when I hear tales about those who quickly lose their mobility, I'm learning to say to myself, *This is their story, not mine.* I remind myself to try to be present for Ingrid, to be a friend to her instead of worrying about my own health.

I offer my hard-earned insight. "Ingrid, your mom probably spent the last ten to twenty years frustrated with the limitations of her body. But she's free from that damaged shell now. Her spirit can do whatever it wants."

She exhales. "It makes me feel better to hear that," she says.

Ingrid and I stay on the phone for more than an hour. She talks to me about what it was like to grow up at the hands of an abusive, psychologically unstable mom. Her mother was institutionalized many times and diagnosed with various psychological illnesses—everything from bipolar disorder to schizophrenia. It sounds like a more extreme version of my own story. I, too, have collected a number of psychological diagnoses over the years as doctor after doctor listened to my odd, unexplainable physical complaints and always deemed my symptoms all in my head. "It must be psychosomatic," was their favorite explanation for years. Even the time my entire body went tingly and numb for six months when I was 23, they claimed "there's nothing organically wrong with you."

After nearly fifteen years of this constant dismissal, I felt somewhat vindicated when my multiple sclerosis diagnosis was finally declared. On the day that San Francisco neurologist pulled up pictures of my brain on a computer and showed me the white areas—the scar tissue of lesions—I remember how angry I felt. I had begged at least three previous doctors to do an MRI because of my chronic pain and stiffness, but they refused. After the anger, my mind went to my aunt. I watched her struggle with MS and degenerate into paralysis in just ten short years. A good friend of my mother's had MS, too, and she was wheelchair-bound in her thirties. These were the only two people I knew with the disease, and for both it progressed especially quickly. I remember feeling a deep sense of impending doom. But, as much as the diagnosis scared me, I wanted to call each of those specialists from years past and exclaim, "See, there really is something physically wrong with me, you idiot!"

Just as they had with me, doctors and psychiatrists prescribed drug after drug to Ingrid's mother for years, until she decided to stop taking any psych meds and turned to self-medicating with alcohol and marijuana. That part sounded very familiar, too. At some point, Ingrid's mom left her father, found another love, and had a few happy, stable years before her MS diagnosis brought her life crashing down.

"Her MS progressed so quickly, it was a shock to us all," Ingrid says. "She was in a wheelchair within a decade and then took to her bed for the final ten years of her life." During this time, Ingrid labored to repair their relationship by making regular visits to her mother's home in England.

It was during one of those visits that Ingrid forgave her mother.

"I was feeding her grapes in bed—she loved plump sweet red grapes—and after swallowing one, she became very serious and said, 'I abused you. I'm so sorry.' It was so weird—just came out of nowhere. I had often wished that one day she would acknowledge the things she did to hurt me and apologize, but never expected it. From that moment on she was my mother again and that was all that mattered. I did my best to care for her."

"Ingrid, your mom loves you so much," I emphasize as I listen to Ingrid sob on the other end of the phone. "You're

grieving right now, but under the tears I can hear your gratitude for the peace you found together."

A long, weighty sigh escapes from Ingrid. There is a final
last rush of tears and then I hear her begin to contain her
sadness by taking three short breaths. I sit silently for a few
seconds and wait for her to calm.

"Thank you for listening," Ingrid says quietly. There's a
bit of shuffling on the other end as she shifts in her seat and
checks her watch. Her voice brightens a bit as she says, "Oh,
look at the time! Here I've chatted your ear off . . . Shall we
still get a bite? I can come pick you up."

To my surprise, I don't feel tired anymore. I am happy to
say yes.

Ingrid pulls up in a cute little black convertible and
honks. I move slowly down the stairs to the car, where I'm
greeted by her adorable dog, a blond Pomeranian sporting a
hot pink collar sparkling with rhinestones. Ingrid is wearing
a blue scarf tied over her chin-length brown hair. As she
helps me into the car, she hands me a couple of black-and-
white photos, old pictures of her mother.

"I thought you'd like to see what me mum looked like,"
she says, smiling.

In the photo, Ingrid's mom is about my age—mid-thir-
ties—and is pretty in a restrained, British way. She looks exactly like Ingrid. When I tell her this, Ingrid says through a
chuckle, "I know, right? I get me good looks from her."

She drives us to Urth Café, a legendary L.A. health food
joint. I eat a delicious tostada and order a piece of sugarless
chocolate cake to go.

After she drops me off, I settle in to watch TV. When

Mark gets home, I decide I will give him the cake as my gift for the day. Though I really want it myself, he has a huge sweet tooth and I love making him happy. *Maybe I could sneak a little piece off before I give it to him,* I think. But I don't.

"I brought you a piece of chocolate cake from the restaurant," I tell him, and he breaks into a grin.

"This looks fantastic! Thank you so much," he says, and digs in. I watch him enjoying the treat and realize that the cake is just a bonus gift. Listening to Ingrid and giving her some compassion was the real gift I offered today. "Gratitude keeps your heart open" was one of Mbali's lessons, and I feel it deeply tonight.

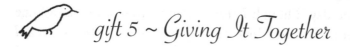 *gift 5 ~ Giving It Together*

After less than a week of giving, despite my early skepticism, there's no denying that something intangible has relaxed inside me. Last time I spoke with Mbali I tried to explain this to her, but she already understood. "It's weird. It's like I'm being supported everywhere I look," I told her. "And the more I give little things, the easier it's become for me to accept assistance and love from others. Instead of being tied up in knots all the time." Mbali had seen this effect many times and wasn't surprised.

"You did something very brave by finally making a choice to answer the call to give your gifts, Cami," she said. "It is a profound moment in all of our lives when we can let go of control and surrender to something bigger."

When I hung up I felt proud to know her. And after giving only four gifts, I have even begun to feel a little proud of myself, something I haven't felt in a very long time.

Today is Easter Sunday. Habib is meowing to be fed, so I follow her to the kitchen. As I pour the kibble into her bowl, I start to think of all the people who could benefit from the giving challenge, as I have. A seed of an idea takes hold, and I start to play around with it.

What if everyone started giving one small thing each day? How different would our world look?

I scratch Habib behind the ears. Her brother, Abu, a huge black cat who is less than graceful, rambles in and begs for equal treatment. So I pet him until he loses interest and begins to lap up water from his yellow ceramic bowl.

What would happen if thousands . . . or even millions of people committed to give away 29 gifts in 29 days?

The spring equinox just passed. It's the time of rebirth and renewal. Crocuses are bursting through thawing snow in other parts of the country, and women are breaking out their white shoes and floral prints. It's the perfect time to start imagining what a movement like this could do on a grand scale.

I decide to do some digging online to see if anything similar already exists. I find www.helpothers.org and immediately fall in love with their Smile Card campaign. People can order little cards that say "Smile. You've been tagged." You're supposed to do or say something nice for another person, then give them the card and encourage them to pass on a good deed to someone else. The website calls it a game of "Pay-It-Forward Tag" and says that more than 450,000 Smile Cards and been delivered to people. Amazing.

I lean back and stretch my arms over my head. I have a lot to be grateful for, starting with my husband, who's been forced to take on the daunting responsibility of walking through life with me. Mark's brown eyes remind me of my dad's and were one of the first things that attracted me to him. His energy is very relaxing—when he enters a room, everyone takes a deep, refreshing breath. He's such a social guy—extremely outgoing, unlike me. I am often shy and hard to get to know.

Mark was the first person I dated who was willing to pry me open and accept what he saw inside. With my depression, addiction, and intimacy issues, that wasn't always a pretty sight. The first time I met him, I was fresh out of drug rehab and attending an addiction support group meeting. Mark was leading the meeting that night and told his story to the crowd. He was so articulate and funny. I introduced myself after the meeting just to say hello. I was in no condition to start dating anyone. I was brand-new to this group, and he was really kind to me. The following week we sat next to each other, but only because we were both late and those were the only seats left.

An entire year went by during which I didn't see him or think about him. Then one evening I was heading into an Indian restaurant in my neighborhood to meet a friend and Mark entered at the exact same time. We bumped into each other in the doorway. It sounds so cliché, but everything seemed to stand still as we stared at each other for this quiet, peaceful moment before the world around us started moving again.

"You look familiar," I said.

"So do you," he answered, but it took a while for us to realize why. Mark finally figured it out, then he ordered some food to go and took a seat. We chatted as he waited. "So the last time I saw you, you were shaking and baking," he said, joking about my fresh-out-of-rehab state.

"Yeah. I wasn't exactly human yet. I've come a long way in the last year."

He was 39—eight years older than me—and he seemed so put-together compared to the less-mature guys I usually dated. His black, button-down shirt had clearly been professionally ironed, the collar and cuffs starched.

We chatted for a few more minutes, and when his order was ready, Mark got up to leave. I felt a sudden panic overtake me. It had been a year since I last saw him, and it was clear he was going to walk out of the café without asking for my phone number. "Hey," I said as he stood up, "I should give you my card and you should call me." I wasn't willing to risk not seeing him again. Thank God he got my not-so-subtle hint and called the next day. It turned out we lived only four blocks apart.

Poor Mark—I needed to take it *very* slowly because this felt so different from previous relationships I'd been in, and I'd just broken up with yet another man who I decided wasn't "the one." I knew there were real feelings with Mark and wanted to make sure we took our time before jumping into a physical relationship. After three weeks of dating, he turned to me one night after we ate dinner at his house. "Can I kiss you?" he asked politely. There was a fire burning in the hearth and the lights were down low. It was the perfect setting for our first kiss.

"I'm not ready yet," I replied nervously, "but I'm really glad you asked."

He cracked up into hysterical laughter at my response. "Okay," he said. "I'll ask again another time."

I called my mother the next morning and said, "I think I met the man I'm going to marry."

I snap out of my reverie when I hear Mark get out of bed and shuffle sleepily down the hallway. He stops outside my office door and looks shocked when he sees me sitting at the computer. For months he has found me in one of two places: horizontal in our bed or horizontal on the living room couch with TV remote in hand.

"Babe. What are you doing?" he asks, rubbing his eyes.

"Just a little research."

"Well, I'm glad to see you starting to act a little more like yourself." He turns and drifts into the bathroom. I bounce in my seat to Blondie's "The Tide Is High" for a minute, then decide to get some breakfast and prepare for church. I haven't been doing the affirmations Mbali mentioned, so I take a moment and say out loud, "Today I give with abundance."

After we eat and shower, Mark helps me put on an orange cotton sundress and some flowered flats—perfect for Easter Sunday—and we make the short drive to the North Hollywood Church of Religious Science. We started attending services at the church not long after we moved to L.A. because we thought it would be a good place to meet some nice people, which turned out to be true. We hadn't intended to become regulars. Neither of us had attended church since we were teenagers. But when we walked into the sanctuary that first time, we both felt at home.

The Church of Religious Science blesses all paths to God. They see all religions as sacred and true. The art on the walls of the sanctuary are evidence of these beliefs. There are paintings of Ganesh, Shiva, Jesus, Buddha, and even a photograph of the Beatles with the Maharishi and a painting that's a parody of the Last Supper, with Jesus surrounded by

12 "disciples" who include Oprah and John Lennon. Mark is a huge Beatles fan so he knew we were in the right place when he saw that. For me, it just felt good to be in a church that celebrates spirituality rather than religion.

Dr. Mark Vierra, the minister, is in prime form today. I think he actually missed his calling as a stand-up comedian. After some good laughs, we all listen intently as Dr. Mark speaks of rebirth and rejuvenation—perfect themes for me right now.

When the collection plate is passed, Mark and I reach into our wallets and each pull out a dollar. We have been strapped financially for a while now and neither of us feels we can afford to give much. As I'm folding my dollar bill and holding it over my heart for the congregational blessing of gifts, I remember my affirmation from this morning. *Today I give with abundance.* I also recall some advice Mbali gave me. "Try to give away something you think you can't live without—or something that feels scarce."

I open my wallet again and find the $20 bill I've saved to put toward our dinner out later. Mark sees me reach for the larger bill and his eyes bug out of his head for a second, then he shrugs his shoulders as if to say, *What the heck, it's only money.* We both bless the bill and smile as I drop it into the collection plate.

I'm feeling tired at the end of the service, but say yes anyway when Mark asks if I want to go to Santa Monica beach. Getting in the car, I turn on the air conditioner, and we head toward the freeway. Mark reaches over and clicks off the AC, and I turn it back on. He looks at me and flips the knob to "off" again.

"Leave the air conditioner on. It's hot as hell," I grumble. "You know I can't handle the heat." I recently began having problems with heat sensitivity. When I overheat, my whole body starts to tingle uncomfortably, and I experience even more weakness and fatigue.

"Calm down," Mark snips back. "I'm just turning it off until we get on the freeway because running the air conditioner makes the car sluggish."

I sit back and swallow my words, though I want to gripe at him more. *Who gives a shit if we have to build up speed slowly? I want to be comfortable.* Lately it's hard to tell when I'm going to feel patient and when I'm going to be a grump. The last person I should get grouchy with is Mark. Yet I'm beginning to feel agitated, and probably not just because of the damn air conditioner.

We soon arrive at the beach. It's one of those perfect L.A. days. The sky is bright and the water stretches out before us like a rolling blue plain. Mark takes my left arm. I put my cane in my right hand and we walk onto the sand. Mark wants to go down near the water, but I find it hard to walk in the sand and nearly trip and fall several times. After the fourth stumble, I throw down my cane and flop onto the sand, crying and yelling like a petulant 2-year-old.

"I hate this!" I pound both fists into the sand and kick my feet. "I just want to go to the beach and enjoy the day with my husband. Why does everything have to be so hard?!"

The beach is crowded and everyone within earshot turns to stare at me. I see that Mark is really embarrassed and that pisses me off more.

"You don't get it!" I yell at him. "You just don't understand how Goddamn frustrating this is. My life will never be normal again. I can't do the things I want to do anymore! I just hate it."

I dissolve into sobs and Mark quietly spreads out the blanket next to me and sits down. "Come over here and calm down, Cami. People are looking at us."

"Well, you better get used to people looking at us! Don't you think people will look when you're pushing me around in a wheelchair? Don't you think they'll look when I can't control my bowels anymore and shit my pants while we're sitting in a restaurant?"

"You're being melodramatic."

"No, I'm not! That's what happens to people with advanced MS, Mark. I think you're in denial about the magnitude of this diagnosis. You're mister skip-along-like-everything-is-okay all the time." He's a chipper guy. Everything rolls off his back. Sometimes I love that about him, and sometimes it drives me absolutely crazy. *Is his happy-guy mask just a way of covering up his own fear?*

I don't know where this all came from on this beautiful day that started out with me feeling just fine. But now that I've erupted, suddenly I'm completely terrified that Mark will leave me because he can't handle the load he's been saddled with in our marriage. I don't know how he manages to work plus take care of me and everything at home. When we started dating four years ago, I was in the best shape of my life. I practiced yoga and walked all over San Francisco because I didn't own a car. I did Pilates and worked out with a trainer regularly. When Mark asked me to marry him, he was getting a healthy, active wife.

Anytime I voice my fear that he'll leave, Mark looks at me like I'm crazy; like the thought of walking away never crossed his mind. But I have trouble believing it. *Is he just being strong for me? Maybe he's just putting on a strong face?* If the tables were turned, I hate to admit it but I'm pretty sure I would at least be thinking about escaping. It must be so hard for him. *Thank God Mark is so kind. I am lucky to have him.*

"Cami, I'm not stupid. I get it," he says slowly. "But if I spend all my time worrying about how bad things might get in the future, I'll miss the good times we can have right now."

By now, tears are streaming down Mark's face, too. "God, honey, I love you so much, but I can't take much more of this. I'm trying so hard to support you . . . to be here for you . . . but you have been really hard to live with for a long time now."

"I'm sorry," I choke out. "That's why I'm always afraid . . . why I worry . . . that you'll, you know . . ."

"I know," Mark replies. "But I'm not going anywhere."

We both calm down and then lie down with our fingers entwined like we're in junior high. *This is a man I can trust,* I think. *That's why I married him.* I sit back up and watch the waves. Mark begins to snore lazily in the sun.

When the heat gets to me, I wake Mark up. We head back to the boardwalk and sit under an umbrella. I drink some iced tea to cool off and then slip under one of the cold outdoor showers, which helps a lot. As I'm standing under the shower in my cotton dress, I notice two girls roller skating. When I was a kid I used to roller skate every day during the summer.

I get out of the shower and announce, "Honey, I want to go skating!" This is a gift I would like to give myself today.

To try to do something I used to love before MS made life hard.

"Are you crazy? An hour ago you were pitching a fit because you couldn't walk in the sand."

"You can help me. Please. I just want to try it for five minutes."

"I know, but what if you fall and hit your head or break your arm?"

"Pleeeease," I wheedle. "You can hold my waist. We'll only go from here to there." I point to the snack stand 25 yards away.

"Woman, you're crazy. And you're so damn stubborn I know you'll do it whether I help or not!"

Shaking his head, Mark checks out a pair of rental skates for me and helps me get them on. "Seriously, if you fall and hurt yourself . . ."

"I'll be fine," I interrupt.

I stand up and Mark stands behind me, his hands on my waist. I start to roll forward slowly.

"I think it will work better if you hold my hand," I say.

Mark nervously takes his hands off my waist and grasps my right hand. Choppily, I begin to roll forward. My balance improves and by the time we reach the snack shack, I'm laughing out loud and squealing, "Look, I'm doing it!" Just like I yelled to my dad when he taught me to ride a bike in our driveway when I was 6.

I don't want to stop at the snack shack, but I know Mark will freak if I try to go farther so I slow down and sit on a cement retaining wall and Mark puts his arm around me, saying, "Way to go, babe!"

We're both finally smiling. "So do you think that $20 we gave today in church will go out and do good in the world?" I ask Mark.

"Absolutely," he replies. "Especially because we gave it together."

gift 6 ~ A Simple Mantra

Two years ago, just one month after my diagnosis, I had a profound experience in meditation that made me a firm believer that meditation can have a direct positive impact on health.

That morning, I awoke at 3 a.m. from a peaceful sleep, sat straight up and yelled out loud: "The symptoms are the cure!"

This woke up Mark, and I began an elaborate, frenzied explanation of this message and vision from my dream.

"Think about how the MS disease process works," I rambled to him. "My immune cells attack my nerve cells, which exposes the nerve. Immediately my body begins to try and repair the damage by forming scar tissue and growing new neural paths to restore the functions associated with that specific area of the nerve. What if the symptoms are actually coming from this healing process—from my nervous system trying to repair itself?" He stopped me after a couple of minutes and told me I should get out of bed and write what I was telling him. I wondered at the time if this might be a ploy to get me out of the room so he could go back to sleep, but I'm so grateful he told me to record my dream because I often refer back to what I wrote that night.

I spent the rest of the wee hours of that morning alternating between meditating, writing in my journal, and going in and out of a "lucid dream" state—this happens when your body is asleep but you're conscious of the dream and you can manipulate it. During the journaling, I drew a bunch of diagrams of what I saw as my "disease process." While I was in the meditative state, I felt that I was watching what was going on in my body on a cellular level. It was as if I was looking at diagrams in a medical textbook. I could *see* the instant one cell would light up and attack the other. Every time I saw this happen, I would talk to the cells and tell them to stop. Over and over I would watch this process begin and then reverse, knowing that if I could see it, I could change the picture. There wasn't anything frightening about it to me. I felt oddly detached, watching my cells in action.

At the time, my main symptoms were memory problems, blurred vision in my right eye, back pain, and numbness in my hands and "my claw"—which happened when a spasm would leave my fingers curled up.

At some point during my meditation, I fell asleep. When I awoke fully in the morning, I had feeling back in two fingers on my right hand and the vision in my right eye was clear again. A message seemed to resonate in the room around me, telling me over and over: "Feel and experience every symptom. The symptoms are part of the healing process."

I meditated daily for several months after that night. My symptoms leveled out significantly and I began to feel good enough to work part-time. I started my own consulting business, but I didn't respect my body's limits. As the business grew I wore myself out trying to keep up. A new host of symptoms preoccupied me, leaving me in more and more pain. Soon meditation became the furthest thing from my mind. I begged my doctors for drugs and was put on a bunch of new meds. They helped for a while, then we made the move to Los Angeles to improve Mark's voice-acting career opportunities and my health took a major downturn.

This was the deal: Mark's career had reached a plateau. He didn't want to wonder twenty years down the line whether he could have succeeded with more creative and fun work than the commercial stuff he tended to get in San Francisco. Thinking it wouldn't happen in a million years (and being no fan of L.A.), I magnanimously said that if he could get signed by an agent in Los Angeles, we would move there. Three weeks later, he made that happen. I agonized over leaving my fantastic support system, but a promise is a promise. What could I do but make the move with him?

I'd brought along a list of physicians recommended by my doctors in San Francisco, but it turned out that none of them were accepting new patients. So I wound up taking a tour of L.A.'s emergency rooms. This I do not recommend. Before entering one ER I had to go through a metal detector. It looked like a clinic in a Third World country, with people lined up and down the hallways on gurneys. Finally, I found myself with a young ER resident who hadn't been in the system long enough to be jaded. She referred me to Dr. N., the neurologist who began to turn everything around for me. In the meantime, though, I'd leave each ER with a new prescription, on top of the piles of pills I was already taking. No one really seemed to be looking at the whole picture. It's a wonder I wasn't in worse shape than I was.

After the drama at the beach yesterday, I need to keep things simple. Incredibly, each day this week I have had a walk, no matter how short. But yesterday's activities wiped me out. Once I've pushed myself too far, I can feel just-finished-a-marathon tired for days. So now I try to rebalance my energy. The best thing I can do for myself on a day like today is yoga.

I've recently found a wonderful yoga teacher named Eric Small. Eric is in his late seventies, though his body is more well toned than many 40-year-olds'. The only thing that gives away his age is his thinning gray hair. You'd never know it by looking at him or watching him move, but Eric has MS. He has been practicing Hatha yoga for nearly fifty years and has been a student of B. K. S. Iyengar for more than thirty years. He is now an Intermediate Senior Level II Iyengar instructor. Eric has created many progressive programs, like the Optimal Living Program, which I'm a member of, under the guidance of B. K. S. Iyengar for the MS Society in Southern California. He credits Iyengar yoga for his good condition, despite living with MS for half a century. He was the first person to explain to me how deep rest can combat MS fatigue and other symptoms. He regularly teaches me yoga poses I can do at home to restore my energy and peace of mind.

As I lie on the floor, my hips propped on a bolster and my legs resting vertically against the wall, I decide to be still for most of the day. Pushing myself through the fatigue often results in an adrenalin-fueled anxiety that always leaves me even more exhausted by evening, yet unable to sleep.

After the yoga, I realize this is the first time in many weeks that my body is not in nervous system overdrive, but calm and settled. I sit down in my soft meditation chair. It's a club-style chair covered in a modernist print of browns and blues—my signature combination of colors seen all through our house. I plant my feet on the floor and lean back.

Mbali had instructed me to meditate, but I'd been struggling with it. This is the first time I've tried it since moving to Los Angeles four months ago—which may be one of the reasons I have continued to go downhill healthwise.

I sit quietly and picture a small gold ball in the center of my head. I imagine my body and the space around it filling up with bright gold energy. I decide to chant a simple mantra as my gift for the day: "May all beings everywhere, including me, be joyous and free." I sing this 29 times. Though this is an unorthodox choice for a gift, it feels like a powerful offering. Wouldn't our world improve if every person on the planet spent five minutes each day sending out positive intentions for others?

As I open my eyes and stretch in my chair, I feel more peaceful. I settle into bed and decide to call my friend Jeff to tell him about my idea of making a wider movement out of the 29 Gifts. I met Jeff recently at church, and he and his wife, Karen, have become good friends, visiting me in the hospital and stopping by the house now and then on hard days to bring lunch. I snuggle under my down comforter and dial Jeff's number. He answers in a brisk tone that I'm not accustomed to hearing from him.

"Hello."

"Uh, hi, Jeff. It's Cami. Am I calling at a bad time?"

"No, that's okay. I'm just a little frustrated right now. I had a new client booked this morning, and he didn't show up. Didn't even call to tell me he isn't coming."

Jeff is a TV and film director and does one-on-one training to teach up-and-coming directors how to make films.

"It's just so irritating. I give people their first session free. I could have booked a paying client in this spot if I knew he wasn't coming. The guy cost me $200."

"I'm sorry," I say. "I was actually calling to tell you about a new little project I'm thinking about."

"Oh yeah?"

"Yeah. I've been giving a small gift every day to someone, taking a suggestion from a spiritual mentor, and I'm feeling some incredibly positive effects from it. I can't help thinking that if everyone tried this simple thing, they'd have great results, too. What do you think about the notion of starting a giving movement, maybe developing a website for it?"

"Huh. I may not be the best person to talk to. I'm sorry, I'm just not in a very giving mood right now."

I decide not to get deflated by his reaction. "I can tell," I say. "But listen anyway." I go on to tell Jeff about Mbali's prescription and the change I've seen in my outlook in the few days since I've been giving daily. "So I'm thinking, what if we invite other people to give for 29 days and share their experiences—how it changes their lives? I think you should be the first member of the movement."

Jeff's silence tells me that he isn't sold on the concept.

"It's an interesting idea," he says. "Is the point just to give, or will people expect things in return? Maybe the first 29 days should be about giving and the next 29 days should be about receiving."

"Well, one of the premises is that giving and receiving are

naturally reciprocal. That if you put your focus on giving, you will receive gifts back from the universe."

"Hmm. I'll think about it. You caught me on a bad day. I'm still pissed off about this client."

"That's okay. I get that. Think about it, and I'll talk to you about it again another day."

Now I'm feeling daunted. If Jeff, who is one of the most generous people I know, is resistant to giving every day for 29 days, how will I inspire strangers to do it?

Next, I need to call my Aunt Janelle. She's in town visiting, having generously offered to fly in from Nebraska to help clean our apartment—something that hasn't been at the top of the priority list for either Mark or me lately. The bathroom in particular has been embarrassingly neglected. At first I felt guilty accepting her offer to help, but now I'm feeling excited about the prospect of clean grout. I reach her at her hotel and we make plans for her to come over tomorrow.

I hang up and shift my mind back to my gift for the day. Somehow sending out positive energy during meditation doesn't really feel like "enough" to qualify. It hasn't involved direct contact with other people, so now the gift feels like it doesn't really count. But then I recall Mbali saying that the gifts can be simple. Grand gestures aren't necessary.

"When you are overgiving, you are not living in abundance, but in scarcity," she told me. "When you give from a place of service, honesty, and fullness, you are left feeling revitalized. When you give from a place of responsibility and obligation, you negate the gift and nothing changes. You may in fact be left feeling resentful and drained." And then she asked me a question: "What lack are you trying to fill in yourself by overgiving?"

The answer to her question has dogged me since childhood. There is some part of me that never feels like I am enough. Growing up, I was an overachiever. I had to be the best at everything, at any cost. It's not that my parents expected perfection from me—I put the pressure on myself.

My mom says when I was 2, I wanted to tie my own shoes but ended up hurling them against the wall because I couldn't do it. When I was 4, I tore pages out of the "big people" books on the bookshelf because I couldn't read the words yet. At 6, I nearly burnt my right ear off trying to curl my own hair with an electric curling iron. And as a 15-year-old, I once cheated on a big algebra test that I'd prepped all night for, instead of risking a B.

For today, I choose to let perfectionism and frustration go. I allow my gift of sending out good vibes in my meditation to count. I rest and fill my own cup today, rather than force myself to perform more. I spend the day reading a good book and taking a couple of naps. Starting to let go of that old perfectionist way of being is a gift to myself.

gift 7 ~ Small Offerings

Aunt Janelle stands in the dining room wearing her cleaning clothes—a pair of black exercise pants, a white T-shirt, and white sneakers. She sits down in one of my tan fake-suede chairs to remove her shoes.

"Should I clean the bathroom first?" she asks.

"I made a list of the things I can't do myself . . . and the things I hate asking Mark for, since he does so much," I say, laying the list on the dining table with equal parts gratitude and guilt. I try to remember Mbali's words: *Giving opens space for you to receive.*

Written on the little slip of pink paper are: bathroom floor, shower tile and tub, toilet and bathroom sinks. Kitchen counters and cabinets. Kitchen floor.

"I can't believe you flew 1,500 miles to clean my house," I say, giving her a little hug.

"That's what family is for. Besides, I really wanted a break from the cold. It's nice to see some flowers blooming. The ground is still frozen in Omaha. And at least there's only one bathroom to clean here—I have four! Cleaning bathrooms at home is an all-day job for me."

Though she's my dad's sister, Janelle is only fourteen years my senior. We have always been close. I often helped take care of her three girls before I moved to California.

48

Janelle scrubs away and we occasionally holler conversation from our posts in different rooms, catching up on members of our family.

While Janelle vigorously scours the grout on my bathroom floor with a toothbrush, I return several phone calls, including one to my contact at the large foundation who inquired about a consulting project on Day 1. He tells me the job, a pretty big one from the sound of it, is likely to begin in two months. I'm relieved that I have some time to get back on my feet before we start.

Incredibly, in the past few days, I've received five other consultation requests through my website, all from small business owners or nonprofits who need help generating name and tagline ideas or marketing plans. I leave messages for four, then the last person picks up—my friend Allie, a fellow marketing consultant from San Francisco. She's in the beginning stages of restructuring her own company and needs help with branding, pricing, that kind of thing. She's the perfect first client for getting back to work, and we book an appointment for April 2. Allie knows me well and is familiar with my health struggles, so I can be honest with her if I need to take breaks to rest.

It feels good to know I'll get a check after that meeting. For months, I have contributed nothing to our household financially beyond my meager disability payments. Yet another weight on Mark's shoulders. (I had to leave my job and go on disability benefits a year and a half ago.) I look at my April calendar and plot in spaces to meet with seven more clients. Assuming the four people I just called will want to book, I leave messages for five of my old clients and tell them I'm going to be back to work in April and have a limited number of appointments available. If I fill all of the open spots, I could generate $4,000 in revenue, which would help put a small dent in the large, looming debt Mark and I have accumulated in recent months.

"Done with the bathroom!" Janelle announces. I step in to admire her work. Who knew the grout on the floor was actually white? The shower, floor, and toilet all gleam. She even scraped all the dried paint splatters off the counter and sink.

"Wow," I say to Janelle. "Thanks so much! Now I can take a bath and not feel like I'm soaking in a cesspool."

Janelle smiles. "There *is* something very satisfying about clean grout." Then she heads into the kitchen and does an equally thorough job there. There's not a speck of food splatter left anywhere on the countertops. When she's finished, even my metal canisters sparkle in the sunlight.

"I wish I had more time so I could clean your wood floors. They really need it," Janelle says, running her white-stockinged foot across the floor and raising it to show me the filthy bottom. "I could call my friend and let her know I can't meet her until later."

"No, no! Go. Believe me, you've done enough. The wood floors can wait until Mark feels up to mopping."

Janelle and I decide to go out to lunch and then walk back to her hotel so she can check out and get her rental car. She admires my decoupaged cane on the way and tells me how glad she is to see me up and around.

"Things were really bad for a while," I confide. "I can't believe I'm even walking, but I have to be careful with my balance. I'm actually getting used to it, though."

"It's good that you're doing what you can. You know what they say . . . use it or lose it. You have to work to keep yourself mobile with MS." Janelle is a licensed physician's assistant, so she really understands the truth of this. In addition, my aunt Margo, Janelle's sister-in-law, has a very progressive form of MS and is nearly completely paralyzed from the disease. Janelle and I have both seen firsthand the utter devastation MS can wreak.

We enjoy lunch together, talking about old times and trading a bit of family gossip. Then we say our goodbyes as Janelle heads out of town to spend the night with a friend from college. She'll be flying back to Omaha tomorrow.

One of my favorite spiritual teachers, Lori Del Mar, always says to me, "A closed hand cannot receive." As I watch Aunt Janelle drive off, I realize that she hasn't just given me the gift of a clean house. Accepting her help is a gift. It was challenging for me to say yes and have her come all this way to scrub floors, but I know Janelle feels happy that she was able to help me. It is such a relief to feel my fists unclench and open up to others.

On my way home, I stop in a corner store to pick up some juice. I lean back against a wall to rest a moment before entering and am overpowered by the smell of sweat and alcohol. Ten feet away, there's a large man resting against a dumpster, holding out his hand in a silent plea for spare change. Instinctively, I avert my eyes and step into the store.

The $5 in my pocket is the last money I can spend until Friday, when Mark and I withdraw our weekly cash allowance out of our dwindling bank account. I make my way into the store, shuffle down the aisle and find my favorite cherry-blueberry juice. As the clerk is giving me change, I stop ignoring the glaring fact that the man in need outside offers a perfect opportunity to give. On the way out, I walk over to him and bend down to put the change in his hand. I look directly into his brown eyes. "It's not much, but I hope it will help you." The coins jingle as 72 cents tumble into his palm.

He smiles at me, pats my hand, and says, "It will. Thanks."

Back at my apartment, I spend most of the afternoon resting. Mark wakes me up for dinner and then takes me to my addiction support group.

I have plans to meet up with Ingrid at this meeting, which is attended by a large British contingent. They even serve tea and "biscuits" instead of the standard coffee and Oreos. I arrive early and save a seat for Ingrid, who is apparently running late. Saving the seat is my second gift of the day—after all, if I don't, Ingrid will have to stand in the back or sit in the overflow room where she'd have to watch the meeting on a television screen. She smiles at me when she arrives, the meeting already under way. At one point, she gets called on to share and I listen intently as she describes how she's still overwhelmed with grief for her mother. As Ingrid sobs uncontrollably, I reach into my purse and pull out some tissues and a bottle of water. I hand them to her when she is done talking. A wave of gratitude washes over her face, and she stops crying long enough to smile. "Thanks, love," she says softly as she twists the cap off the water. She takes a gulp, then wipes her tears with the tissue.

It's clear to me that often the simplest gifts carry the most meaning. The small gestures that show people you care. A kind word instead of keeping quiet. The smile you choose to break free for someone you don't know. The sincere gratitude you express to someone for assisting you in some way. The spare pennies—or spare tissues—you choose to pass along to someone who needs them more than you do. I've been giving small gifts every day for a week now, but in the scheme of things I feel way ahead.

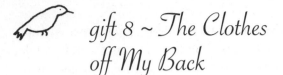

gift 8 ~ The Clothes off My Back

"Okay. I'm in," Jeff says.

"Huh?" I'm not with the program yet. I've been having yet another nap.

"Oh sorry, did I wake you? I just called to let you know I'm in for the giving project. I started yesterday."

I work my way to a sitting position, almost dropping the phone in the process. "I'm so happy you're saying yes!" I beam. "I figured I'd never be able to start a giving movement if I couldn't even recruit you."

Jeff laughs. "Sorry. I was just in a bad mood that day. I think this is a really great idea. I'm curious to see what will happen for me."

"What do you hope will happen?"

"Well, I don't really have expectations, but I hope giving frees up some energy in my work life. I haven't made much money lately, but the writer's strike is finally settled so maybe some gigs will come my way." The Writer's Guild has been on strike for months now, which has put a halt to much of the entertainment industry work in Hollywood.

"It's certainly possible. I've already booked two new clients this week! Things are definitely heating up."

"I hope so. Karen would be thrilled if I made some money."

Jeff and I have commiserated before about how hard it is on our spouses when business slows for us. Jeff's wife, Karen, works as a graphic designer—a job she doesn't love—to help pay the bills. She really wants to go freelance and pursue her career as an artist, but hasn't felt safe making the leap because they rely heavily on her income.

"Mark has talked about taking a part-time job at UPS to help pay the bills," I tell Jeff. "I really don't want him to do that."

"Yeah," Jeff says. "I'd love to start bringing in steady cash so Karen can make some changes for herself. But it feels wrong to go into this giving experiment expecting to get money in return. I'm just going to focus on giving each day and see what happens."

"That's what I'm hoping people will do. I've had fun with it so far. Today is Day 8 for me." I recap the gifts I've given.

"I want to try not to give money. I'd rather give my time and talents to others . . . or use this as an opportunity to pass on some things I'm not using anymore. Do you plan what you're giving each day?" asks Jeff.

My first inclination actually had been to plot out the whole experiment and line up the 29 things down my hallway—maybe to give myself some illusion that I can control what happens.

"No, that goes against the spirit of this. I just go through each day and remain open to opportunities where I can give. So far it's been pretty easy. Oh, and Jeff," I add, "it's funny, but though you want to be of service to others, this is really about shifting the energy around yourself so that you can learn to be grateful for your day, for your life. It reminds you that you're part of something bigger and that you do have gifts to offer the world."

It feels good being able to pass along Mbali's words. "Give your gifts with an open heart," I went on, "without any expectation that you will receive something in return." I told him about the affirmations and the meditations, too—and the motivator, if he needed it: "Try not to skip a day once you begin. The ritual needs to gather its own momentum, and you really should start again at Day 1 if you miss a day, to allow the energy to build again."

By the time I hang up, I'm giddy. I have my first recruit! Now I need to think about setting up a website that will allow me to connect easily with the people who say yes. My friends are spread out all over the country and I want us all to be able to communicate. I've found an online tool called Ning that makes it easy to build your own social network. People can join by filling out a profile, and each person gets a blog—where I'm hoping they'll share stories about the gifts they're giving. I type an e-mail to 29 friends, inviting them to join me on the site, which I have up and running in no time:

Dear Friends,

Most of you know I've been having a really hard time with my MS for several months now. Thanks to all of you who have sent cards and prayers, especially during my last hospital stay. I'm happy to report that I've begun to feel better. I recently decided to take a suggestion from one of my spiritual teachers that has helped. The suggestion is to give away a gift a day for 29 days.

So far, I've given seven small gifts and have been amazed at the wonderful, unexpected things that have come back to me. I've started walking again and have managed to go on a short walk with my cane every day for the past week!

Because you're one of my friends who is a natural giver, I thought you'd be interested in doing this with me.

We can use the site I've set up at www.29Gifts.org to share stories about our giving experiences.

Please feel free to forward this e-mail to anyone you think would find this fun. I love you all!

Cami

My phone rings later in the afternoon and it's my friend Eve, one of my friends who received the message. She tells me she loves the idea and plans to start her giving next week.

"Would you be willing to give a gift to the giving challenge?" I ask her.

"What do you need?"

"I want the website for the project to have a custom design—something cooler than the template site I put up today. I'm wondering if you'd be willing to do the design and programming. Um, for free."

This takes chutzpah. Eve is a first-class, self-taught web geek and an extremely busy person. I've hired her to create a number of websites for my clients. She always gives me "friend" rates, but she's never done anything for me gratis. And this could be thousands of dollars' worth of work. She has skills that I need, but I realize I'm skirting dangerously close to the outer boundaries of friendship.

"Sure," she says without hesitation, and moves right on. "I actually was calling to ask you for a little help with something. I'm going to South Africa to teach as a volunteer this summer and I need to raise $10,000 to fund my trip. I've written a letter to send to my family and friends and was hoping you'd edit it for me."

I'm relieved to have a chance to reciprocate Eve's kindness in advance. "Of course. E-mail it to me and I'll look at it tomorrow." That'll be my gift for the day. "But you're getting the short end of this deal. I'll probably spend an hour on your letter, but you'll spend about twenty hours on my site."

"Good thing I love you."

"Yeah, good thing," I laugh.

"So how did you meet this medicine woman? What's her name again?"

"Mbali," I say, and I go on to tell Eve the story of how Mbali used to be our neighbor in Oakland.

When Mark and I moved to a smaller place in San Francisco to save money and be closer to my doctors, I remember thinking that I probably wouldn't ever see Mbali again. She would join the ranks of the many people who I briefly connected with, but with whom I never had the chance to develop a fully formed friendship. Instead, within weeks of settling into our new cracker-box of an apartment, I received an e-mail from my friend Angel, a meditation teacher whom I had just begun working with.

Her email announced that Mbali was going to be the featured guest at Angel's "healing salon" the following week.

That's a gathering of people who do different types of body work, meditation, and such who get together once a month with a speaker who demonstrates or discusses their work. Mbali would be demonstrating Cowrie Shell Divinations. What a serendipitous surprise! I had no idea that Angel knew Mbali, but it turns out they had been colleagues for over a decade.

Eve's voice interrupts my story for a moment. "So did you go to the healing salon?"

"Of course. I was curious. I had no idea what a Cowrie Shell Divination was."

When I walked into Angel's living room, Mbali was sitting cross-legged on the floor with a large cloth spread out in front of her. Hand-painted symbols covered the cloth. Odd shapes. Footprints. Handprints. A compass-looking thing. I wasn't sure what to think. Mbali was really surprised to see me show up at the salon, and we greeted each other warmly. The polished, professional garb I was used to seeing Mbali wear when we carpooled to work was gone. Instead, she was wearing tribal patterns, big chunky tribal jewelry, a shell-encrusted belt, and an African-style head wrap with a porcupine quill sticking out of it. She wore a leather medicine pouch around her neck. Angel introduced her as a medicine woman, the first time I'd heard that title. I gathered in a circle with seven other women and settled in to watch Mbali do a Cowrie Shell Divination for Angel.

Mbali began chanting a lovely song, welcoming all of us and our ancestors to the circle. She removed the leather pouch from around her neck and pulled out three African cowrie shells, which she carefully placed to her right side.

She opened a basket next to her and then another pouch. She poured a pile of crystals, shells, and rocks in the center of the compass-style drawing in the middle of her cloth. Then she reached into a Ziploc bag and added a handful of ash to the pile. "For protection," she told us in her fluid voice.

Protection from what? I couldn't help but wonder.

Mbali opened yet another basket and pulled out several items, including a real chicken claw that, by the looks of it, had been severed from its owner some time ago. After the ceremony was complete, Mbali turned to Angel and asked, "What is your question?"

Angel told Mbali about her dream from the night before. In the dream, Angel's deceased father walked up to her and handed her an infant and then walked away. "I want to know what that dream meant," she said. "Does my father have a message for me?"

Mbali clarified. "So your question is, 'What is the message your father intended to deliver in this dream?'"

"Yes," Angel responded quietly.

Mbali proceeded with the divination, which seemed similar to a psychic reading, but using different tools. She asked Angel many questions and used her cowrie shells to give direction to the reading, like a tarot card reader does. Angel learned that her father, who was incredibly violent with her mother when she was pregnant with Angel, was giving Angel back her childhood by handing her that baby. "Your father wants to tell you that though there was a lot of trauma and abuse in your life as you grew up, your parents conceived you in love," Mbali said in a mesmerizing tone. "He is offering to reconcile with you. He wants your forgiveness."

As soon as the evening wrapped up, I approached Mbali and scheduled a time to come see her for my own divination the following week.

I've been talking so long on the phone that my ear is numb so I have to switch the receiver to my other side. "So did you go?" Eve asks.

"Yes, I showed up, but the appointment unfolded very differently than I expected."

I wasn't feeling well when I arrived at Mbali's, and she was concerned that my energy might be too depleted to do a divination. We sat down across from each other and she sang her opening invocation chant. She pulled out her cowrie shells from the pouch. "Is it safe to proceed?" she called out, loudly. She threw the shells and all three landed face down. She asked three more times, and three more times all three shells landed face down. "I'm sorry. That is a very clear no," she said to me. "We can't proceed with a divination, but instead I'd like to perform a sweep for you."

"A sweep?"

"It's an energy clearing. A healing. Do you give me permission to move forward?"

I have been a student of other healers who do energy-based healing. Conventional allopathic Western medicine, in fact, is one of the only philosophies that *doesn't* incorporate energy theory—Eastern, Chinese, Ayurvedic, homeopathic, massage, even chiropractic, all have a fundamental understanding that the body is an energy system and that there's a benefit to treating the body at an energy level. Energy patterns can get out of balance and cause blockages, or you can have too much energy flowing through areas. These imbalances manifest as illness. The goal of such treatment is to reestablish balance.

"Sure," I said. One thing I've learned working with healers over the years is that the techniques are irrelevant. What matters is the intention of the healer and I trusted Mbali held pure intentions for me. She spread a pale green sheet out on her living room floor and asked me to lie down on my back. Then she went to her fridge.

"Luckily, I went to the farmers' market today and they had quail eggs. I'll use three of them for you."

Quail eggs?

One at a time, Mbali rolled each egg along the front of my body, over each foot, leg, my belly, chest, and face. I turned over, and she did the same thing on the back. Then she cracked the eggs into a bowl.

"What will you do with them?" I asked, nodding to the eggs as she helped me sit up to face her.

"I'll bury them in my back yard. I need to put you in the shower now," she told me. "Go into the bathroom, remove your clothing and get into the shower with the water as hot as you can tolerate," she instructed. "I'll be in there soon to complete the sweep."

I did what she said and heard her enter the bathroom as I was standing under the water. It was freezing at first, then it came out in a scalp-scalding burst. I spat expletives as the searing water hit my head.

"Are you all right?" I heard Mbali ask.

"Sorry," I said. "I'm okay."

"I'm going to pour something over your head now. Rub it into your scalp."

I heard the shower curtain move and Mbali's cocoa-colored arm reached in.

"Turn with your back to me," she said.

I turned around and was relieved to feel cold liquid hit my scalp. A flowery scent mixed with the steam in the shower. Mbali left the room. I rubbed the scented liquid in as she told me to, turned off the water, dried off and dressed.

I stepped into the living room and sat down on the small sofa. Mbali sat on a pillow on the floor in front of me.

"I have instructions for you for a ritual I want you to do within the next week. It's a 'prescription' of sorts," she said and went on to explain. "Take off the clothing you're wearing as soon as you get home and put it into a plastic bag. Go out into nature and make an offering of a quarter, a small bottle of alcohol and some flowers. You're offering these things to your ancestors. Ask for any guidance you feel you need from your ancestors.

"Sometime in the next seven days, you will meet a homeless man. Buy lunch for him and offer him seven dollars in cash. You will know the person when you see him. You will likely pass by him and then need to turn around and go back or go out of your way somehow to give him your offerings. After you have done all of this, give away the clothing you're wearing today. Throw away the undergarments. And then you can come back in two weeks for your divination."

"But this is a brand new shirt and pair of jeans!" I whined. "And this bra cost $90. It's a year old, but still in great shape. Today is the first time I've worn the shirt and jeans."

Mbali smiled, entertained. The freckles sprinkled across her nose and cheeks glinted a bit in the sunlight streaming through her living room window. "It's up to you if you want to follow these suggestions. Your choice," she said in her British accent.

I left Mbali's house baffled. Something profound had happened to me in that room. I'm not sure what it was, but it had a powerful effect on me. I knew I would be back to work with Mbali again.

Through the phone, I hear Eve's snicker. "Oh, no, not your fancy bra! Did you do it?" she asks.

"Sort of," I respond, and I go on to tell Eve the rest.

I got home that day and bagged the clothes, tucking them into a corner in my closet. The next day I went out to Lands End, a beautiful trail that runs along the Pacific coast. It's my favorite spot in San Francisco, soaring ocean cliffs alternating with wooded areas and wonderful ocean views. On a plateau, at the base of one cliff, was a circular labyrinth made of stones. I walked the labyrinth and in the center made the offerings Mbali suggested. I left a quarter, a small open bottle of Absolut vodka (my old favorite drink), and three little purple wild flowers that I picked along the way. I paused for a while and meditated. I asked my ancestors for help silently. *Help me understand the cause of my MS and heal myself. Please take away my fear and anxiety and reignite my creativity. Please help Mark and me thrive together.*

The following day I was walking down Valencia Street on

my way home after an acupuncture appointment. The sky was spitting that annoying rain that constitutes winter in Northern California. I was angry that I forgot my umbrella. I should have known better after ten years in San Francisco. I was soaking wet within a few blocks.

I passed a man lying sprawled on the ground, clearly sick and so skinny every bone protruded at painful-looking angles. His dark eyes were sunk into his coffee-colored skin, surrounded by puffy purple circles. A cane lay near him. I passed him as I always did when I saw homeless people, looking the other way so I didn't make eye contact and then have to apologize and shake my head to the hand asking me for money. I walked the remaining three blocks, and just as I inserted the key into my front door, I realized, *That is the man I'm supposed to make my offerings to.* I let out an exasperated huff. *Why didn't I think of this sooner? I don't want to spend another thirty minutes in the rain.* But I turned away from my door anyway and walked back in my slow, shuffling gait.

I went into a Mexican restaurant and bought three tacos to go and a large bottle of water with my ATM card. The restaurant didn't give cash back, so I walked another two blocks to a corner store where I found an ATM machine, took out $20, then bought a candy bar so I could break the bill. I put the candy bar into the bag with the tacos and returned to the man. I bent down because he was still lying on the sidewalk. His brown eyes couldn't focus, and the whites were yellow and bloodshot. I could see a tell-tale AIDS lesion on his neck. *This man is dying,* I thought.

I handed him the bag and said, "I brought you lunch."

Then I handed him the $5 and two $1 bills rolled up and said, "This is also for you."

He took the money and put it into his pocket. "Can you put the bag down here?" he asked, patting the ground in front of him. Three of his front teeth were missing. He reached for his cane and struggled to stand. I instinctively grabbed his free elbow to steady him. Once he was on his feet, the man reached out and touched my left shoulder with his free hand. Tears leaked from his tired eyes. "Thank you so much," he said to me. "God will bless you for your kindness."

A warm wave went through me, and I smiled at him. "Thank you. I hope you like tacos."

He broke into a laugh much heartier than I imagined him capable of. "I do. Very much."

"Good. Enjoy your lunch. Get out of the rain and have some hot tea. You shouldn't be out here in the damp cold."

"I will. Have a nice day," said the man as he reached down to pick up the bag of food.

I watched him walk into the coffee shop next door, then I ambled home slowly, feeling grateful that I had a home to go to, shelter from the rain, and food in my kitchen. I also felt a glimmer of gratitude that the chronic disease I'm dealing with isn't AIDS. Multiple sclerosis itself is rarely fatal. I'm likely to live a long life, even if I end up impaired. Sometimes it's hard not to feel sorry for myself, but there are certainly worse illnesses to have.

"Wow." Eve is silent for a moment on the other end of the line. "What did you do with the clothes?"

"I decided to keep the $90 bra, but throw away the panties. I kept the jeans and gave away the shirt. You know what's interesting?" I say to Eve.

"What?"

"That day, I thought I had struck a good compromise with myself about the clothing, but looking back now I see not letting go of those material items was me resisting change."

"Interesting. Do you still have the bra and the jeans?"

"Yes. They're actually one of only two pair of jeans I own right now. And the bra is one of three bras I own. I purged when we moved to L.A. and gave away a lot of clothes."

"Hmmm. But two of the items you chose to hold onto were the things Mbali said to give away. What do you make of that?"

"I guess I'm *still* resistant to change," I say and laugh.

Eve and I have been on the phone for over an hour. After I hang up, I go directly to my dresser to get the jeans and the bra. I throw the bra away and toss the jeans into a shopping bag to take to Goodwill. I'm ready to let go. Finally.

gift 9 ~ Thanks, Mama, Thanks

I'm putting together a gift for my mom, for flying out on short notice the week before my medical detox. I write her a thank-you note and package it up with some Korean Citron Tea. The jar of tea actually looks suspiciously like orange marmalade. But once the sticky substance is dissolved in hot water, it transforms into the tastiest tea imaginable. Dr. Kim gave me two jars of it at my appointment yesterday because she knows how much I like it. As I write my mother's address in Kimball, Nebraska, the address where I spent my childhood, I start thinking about that one-stoplight town in western Nebraska. I was the oldest of three girls. Joelle, Deena, and I were usually a handful, yet my mom has always been the most patient and giving woman I know.

She recently allowed an entire family to live in her house for a couple of months because they'd hit hard times. Years ago, after all three of her kids were out of the house, mom invited a teenage girl to move in for almost a year. She had been kicked out by her mother after a fight. My mom donates to lots of charities, gives monthly to her church, and volunteers in her community. She's a giver and always has been. She was a kindergarten teacher for thirty-three years. As far as I'm concerned, anyone who can spend their days with other people's 5-year-olds and then go home and be a loving mother to her own kids deserves sainthood.

My mom and dad have been married almost forty years. Once, when I asked mom for the secret to their long-lasting marriage, she said, "It's very simple. We never break up. No matter what."

My father is also generous. If a family member or friend needs help, Larry Walker is often the first guy they call. To support our family, he owned a pharmacy and, after filling prescriptions six days a week, he somehow managed to find time for a farming business on the side. Farming is in my dad's blood—his parents, grandparents, and great-grandparents were all farmers. And though my grandparents insisted their kids go to college, my father never lost his love for the land. His hard work paid off, and he sustained our family well over the years. We weren't rich, but we always had what we needed and then some. One thing I can appreciate now is that my dad taught my sisters and me the value of a dollar by making us work for anything we wanted. These are old-fashioned Midwestern farm values, and they have served me well.

When I wanted a new bike at age 7, I spent many hours down at the pharmacy—which was also a gift store—helping with menial tasks like wrapping presents and cleaning the stockroom so I could earn $40 to pay for half the bike. My dad's lesson stuck, and I took good care of that bike. I earned its yellow banana seat and the shimmery, metallic ribbons that hung off the handlebar grips.

The thing about my dad is that though he was careful about money, he didn't hoard it. He once put a down payment on a house and co-signed for some family friends who had lost their farm. Granted, this was Nebraska and a house didn't cost much more than a car! But still, how many people would have done such a thing? He also lent college money to a close friend's son. I earned a full-ride academic scholarship, so Dad got off pretty easy with me—that is, until I dropped out right before my senior year to start a web design and multimedia company. I think he would have gladly paid cash to keep me in school, but I couldn't be swayed, so he gave me and my business partner a couple of small loans to help us start our business.

My business partner was a 22-year-old guy I was in love with, and the two of us made just about every mistake possible starting our business. We financed most of the start-up costs for the company on credit cards secured in my name. We hired our friends from school, most of whom weren't designers or programmers. In fact, all of us were just learning the skills we needed as we went along since none of us had any real work experience. We had a lot of fun and even a few successes before it was time to admit failure and walk away.

But I paid a price. At age 23, I had to file for bankruptcy. I remember calling my dad to tell him the extent of the debt I'd amassed, hoping he'd bail me out. But he didn't. He told me to deal with the consequences of my choices and figure out how to get out of the mess myself. At the time, of course, I was just enraged. Now that I'm almost fifteen years older, I can see it as a difficult act of generosity on his part. No father wants to watch his daughter suffer through her mistakes, but letting me take my hard knocks and learn my own lessons was a gift.

There's something else about my memories of Nebraska. I know there is a high incidence of autoimmune disease in the area where I grew up. In my immediate family alone, four out of five of us have autoimmune diseases. My mother has fibromyalgia, one sister has celiac disease and the other has psoriasis. My father is the only one who has escaped with his immune system intact. On my mom's side of the family, her father, her sister, and one of my cousins all have autoimmune conditions as well.

It's big farm country and there were always crop dusters spraying thick clouds of pesticides. It was like a game to us as kids—we'd chase after them on our bikes. I wonder how many of us were chasing our own future diseases on those bike rides? Not only did I grow up where everything we ate was sprayed, but much of the livestock was given growth hormones, so the meat we ate was pretty tainted as well. To add insult to injury, Kimball, Nebraska, was also oil country, so they were constantly drilling. That couldn't have done wonders for our groundwater supply. Two of my childhood best friends had oil wells in their backyards.

The icing on this toxic cake is that during the 1960s, 1970s, and 1980s Kimball was known as "Missile Town, USA," because we were surrounded by underground nuclear missile silos. There was actually a life-size, disarmed Saturn 5 missile smack dab in the middle of our largest city park. After disarmament, we kids used to play in the abandoned silos that were left unsecured, spelunking through the vast cement caverns as we reenacted Indiana Jones–like adventures. Can you imagine the level of radioactivity we were all exposed to over those decades?

Doctors and scientists do not yet know what causes MS or most other autoimmune diseases, though much research has been done. There are three primary causal factors that seem to overlay each other, though: genetic predisposition (which I am clearly blessed with), environmental toxicity (obviously a biggie for me), and unresolved viral activity in the body (which is also a major part of my medical history).

Back to some better memories of my hometown as I put together the thank-you package for my mom. It occurs to me I should enclose one of Mark's recent headshots. He just took some new ones for his acting agent, and the photographer had him dress up as a number of characters. In one of my favorite poses, Mark is wearing a plaid flannel shirt, an unzipped green hooded sweatshirt and a beat-up John Deere cap: the friendly farmer.

I dig around in Mark's office to find a print. God, he looks just like my dad when he was younger! What would Freud say? He's got the same friendly brown eyes, dark hair slightly receding on top, and that half-smile I recall seeing on my father's face a lot. My dad is as Midwest as they come, a real Nebraska man. After studying the photo, I think Mark should be cast as the John Deere spokesman. He definitely looks the part. My mom will get a big kick out of the photo, so I drop it into the box and seal it up.

I start thinking about the possibilities for the giving movement I hope to start. First, a name: I settle on the 29-Day Giving Challenge. I know Eve will come up with a great design. It feels good to think I can share some of the good fortune I've had, and it certainly keeps me from dwelling on the ways MS holds me back. Just as I'm thinking it might be a good idea to clear all this with Mbali before I go any further, my phone rings and it's Mbali herself.

"I'm calling to check in and see how you're feeling," she says.

"Pretty good, I have to say. And I just want to tell you again how affected I've been since I started giving. I'm feeling more positive in general. It's so nice to wake up and be able to think about what's possible instead of how screwed up my life is." As I say it out loud, it takes on even more truth. I'm starting not to be that resentful, angry, frustrated woman anymore. I hope it lasts.

"Yes. You're putting your consciousness on what you have to offer the world instead of what is scarce."

"I really feel that change."

"Try to be conscious if you feel yourself giving out of obligation. If so, you are in scarcity mode. You end up feeling drained and burnt out . . . out of balance. For me a good measure when I'm making a choice to give is to ask myself, will making this offering fuel me, give me energy? If the answer I get from my heart is yes, I know I am offering an authentic gift out of love."

I will keep coming back to these principles. But they make sense to me now, and I can appreciate how a simple daily act can have profound repercussions.

Now on to more practical considerations. This is my opportunity to tell Mbali about my wider designs for a giving movement—and I certainly don't want to move ahead without her approval.

"Mbali, I wonder how you would feel about me trying to reach other people, a *lot* of other people, to join the giving challenge. A giving *movement*."

She is silent for a few seconds.

"What would be your purpose in starting this movement?"

My heart drops, just for a moment. What if she doesn't go for the idea?

"Well," I explain carefully, "my purpose would be to create a revival of the giving spirit among people."

I let this sink in, wondering what's going through her head. "I like that," she finally responds.

"So does that mean I have your permission to move forward with the project? I wouldn't feel comfortable doing anything official about it without your blessing."

"You have my blessing, Cami. Perhaps we can even figure out a way for me to be involved."

"That would be fantastic!" I tell her, and my mind goes to work immediately on how she could contribute her philosophies in a blog.

"By the way," I say before letting her go, "why did you suggest 29 gifts in 29 days? Why that number? I'm curious."

"That is what my teacher suggested to me when she gave me the ritual to do. I'm unsure of the symbolism of the number 29. Maybe it's related to the moon cycle? I could find out for you."

"That's okay," I tell her. "I kind of like the mystery of not knowing for sure."

Mbali and I chat for a bit longer and then sign off. I hang

up feeling very grateful for her blessing and her wise words. And very much needing to lie down.

After a long nap, I still feel tired, like my mind was jogging while I slept. So I move from the bed to the couch and consume some TV, which just drains me more.

Maybe I'll try a walk, I think halfheartedly as I switch off the television and stretch on the couch. Just over a week ago, I walked several blocks two days in a row. But sometimes I can't make it very far and I get scared I'll be stuck somewhere. Then I perk up as an idea sparks. *Why have I never thought of this solution before?* I can walk one lap around my block. If that poops me out, I'll come home. If I still have enough energy, I'll do it again. *Who cares if I just walk around the same block over and over?*

Cane in tow, I head slowly down the steep set of stairs leading to my front door. I begin to feel dizzy and off-balance so I sit down on a stair to rest. Then I descend the rest of the stairs the safest way I can: scooting down slowly on my butt, one stair at a time. Not graceful, but safe.

Outside, the sunlight is nearly blinding and my progress feels incredibly slow, but when I loop back in front of my house, I'm feeling steady on my feet so I make another round. Then two more. During the fifth lap, I nearly fall a couple of times, but I make it back to the porch in one piece and then sit down and rest before climbing back up the stairs.

While I'd lain around for months, pissed off that I couldn't leave the house, I'd never been able to see the possibilities that were there all along, outside my own front door.

gift 10 ~ Bright Ideas

The physical rehabilitation group I joined not long after arriving in L.A. is cheerfully named the Optimal Living Program. I missed the last two meetings because I was in the hospital, where I was certainly far from living optimally. Today is my first day back. I was in so much pain the last time I attended that I spent most of the session flat on my back, crying.

I bring a book that I read in the hospital to give to Beth, one of the members of the group. She mentioned at the last meeting I attended that she loves reading, especially complex mysteries, but had recently been having trouble following the plots. One of the suggestions from the occupational therapists was to try reading different types of books that aren't as complicated. The book I tuck into my tote bag, *The Big Book of Bright Ideas* by Sandra Kring, fits the bill. It's a light-hearted story about the healing power of friendship, and I hope Beth likes it.

Mark drives me to the building where the meeting is held, and I slowly work my way inside. I am the last person to arrive, and when I walk in, the four therapists and six participants all light up with smiles.

"Cami! I'm so happy to see you up and around," says Fran, one of the patients.

Several others give me friendly greetings as I settle into a chair. *How nice to be welcomed like this.*

Everyone wants to know how the hospital stay was, so I give them a few highlights. I tell them about the nightmarish detox, the fellow inmates in the asylum, and how good it felt to get the hell out of there after eight days. I can't really explain what it feels like when substances your body has grown to depend on are yanked away, so I don't try.

"I made this cane while I was there," I say, proudly holding it up like we're all in first grade playing show-and-tell.

"I was admiring it when you walked in," says one of the therapists. I pass the cane around the room for everyone to examine.

I turn to Beth. "I brought you a book you might like. It's not a mystery, but it's a really wonderful story."

Beth thanks me and then the therapists begin our session. Today Beth, Fran, and I are going to be in a discussion group with one of the therapists. We're going to look at photos of our homes so we can get recommendations on how to make the space safer and more functional. I'm a little bummed that I'm not assigned to a group with Lauri, because she's my closest friend there, but it will be good to get to know Fran and Beth better. We look at my pictures first, beginning with my living room and dining room. The therapist suggests removing all of our area rugs because of the tripping hazard.

"I'll think about getting rid of them," I say. To me, plain hardwood floors feel cold. Plus, the rooms in our house are large with high ceilings, so the rugs cut down on echoes. Without them, I'm afraid the place won't really feel like a home. I know this is silly—why risk tripping and hurting myself for acoustics and aesthetics? But I know myself well enough to be pretty sure the rugs will stay.

The bathroom tour isn't much fun either. The therapist suggests we install grab bars in our shower and around our toilet so I can get on and off the can and in and out of the tub without falling down. I feel the heat rise into my face and know I'm blushing deep red.

"But then everyone who goes into my bathroom will know I'm a gimp!" I blurt.

"Do you want to be safe or protect your ego?" asks Beth bluntly.

"Honestly, I think my ego is more important to me right now." It's not easy to admit this out loud. Anyone I know well enough to invite into my home would surely know I have MS. But if things look normal on the outside, I can play a game with myself that they are normal on the inside.

"I'm just not ready to give in to this disease," I say by way of explanation. "I know you guys think it's crazy, but you've both had two or three decades to accept what's happening to your bodies. I've only been living with the reality of MS for two years. And part of me still believes I can make it stop. I know medical science has no answers for me, but I still believe there are answers out there somewhere."

"Cami, the sooner you accept the limitations of your MS, the easier your life will be," says Fran. There is truth in her words, but I don't want to hear it.

The ideas they give me for changes to the kitchen are easier to swallow, and I agree to address everything they bring up. I don't mind adding pulls to the drawers and cabinets because some days my hands are so stiff and weak I can't open them. Besides, these can be pretty and won't mark me as disabled. They recommend creating stations in the room. The blender and juicer could be in one area, along with other items I use regularly. This way I'm not wasting energy wandering all over the kitchen to gather the things I need each morning and then putting them all away. I could also get a rolling cart so I can put dishes and food on it and roll it around the room or into the dining room instead of making several trips. It comes down to energy conservation—maximizing efficiency so I can use my energy for the highest-priority tasks in my life.

The last space they look at is my entryway. Examining my picture, they comment on how dark and steep the stairwell looks.

"I'm worried you'll trip because you can't see well and fall down those stairs," says Fran.

"I know. I worry about that, too. And this photo was taken with the light on. You should see it in the dark."

"That's not safe," says Fran.

"My landlord isn't a big spender. I don't think she'd wire in another light fixture."

"I have an idea," says Beth. "Get some rope light and string it along the baseboards all the way up the stairs. Rope light is cheap. It's just little white lights strung along an electrical cord, encased in clear rubbery tube."

"Brilliant!" I exclaim. "I can't believe I never thought of something like that. I have lots of white Christmas lights I could use, so I don't have to spend any money at all."

When we're done looking at the photos of my house, we

review Fran's and Beth's photos. Since both of them have been dealing with mobility issues for some time, there aren't many additional suggestions offered to them.

We all head on to the physical therapy portion of our day. My team of three physical therapy students are thrilled to see me walk into the room. They all admire my cane and listen to my tales of hospital woe. Then we do some stretching and balance exercises. They have me stand on a small rubber platform that has a slightly rounded bottom and surround me as I attempt to keep my balance for a few seconds at a time. I tell them that I went roller skating for about 25 yards a few days ago and they all cheer and pull their clipboards out to note it on my progress report. I also tell them that I intend to return to my yoga class the following Monday, which they note as well.

Mark picks me up when the program ends for the day. As we're getting into the car, I notice that Lauri is sitting in her scooter waiting for her van service for people with disabilities. It is really hot outside, so I go into the nearby snack bar and buy her a cold bottle of water to drink while she waits. The van is way behind schedule, and she's frustrated. I assure her that we'll wait with her until it arrives. She looks relieved. Once or twice the van never showed, and if that happens today, we can give her a ride. After ten more minutes the van pulls up, and the driver helps Lauri inside. Now I have given two gifts for the day, the book for Beth and waiting to make sure Lauri makes it home safe. Plus the bottle of water.

As Mark and I drive home, I tell him about the day and the changes we're supposed to make to the house. I think he's relieved to hear that there are some simple things we can do to make life safer for me. *He must worry about me when he isn't home to help me take a shower or get up and down the stairs,* I realize. When we get home, he gets right to work.

I watch Mark string white Christmas lights up the entry-way baseboards and plug them in to illuminate the dark stairwell. He hammers a little nail into the baseboard every couple of feet to anchor them in place. It looks kind of fes-tive, and I'll never have to worry again about that dim stair-way being responsible for any falls. Then I sit on a stool while he makes some efficiency upgrades in the kitchen.

"Let's go shopping this weekend for some cabinet pulls I can maneuver easily," I suggest. "And even the safety bars for the bathroom. You know, these things really will make my life easier. I just have to get past the feeling that I'm giving in to the MS."

Mark looks visibly relieved that I'm agreeing to these changes. I feel relieved, too. For a long time the MS was the only thing I could think about, leaving no room in my head for a peaceful thought. If I work with it instead of against it, I just may free myself up for all kinds of things.

Mark smiles at me and comes over to give me a hug. I hold him close and take a slow and easy breath.

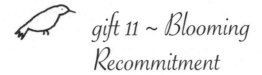

gift 11 ~ Blooming Recommitment

I've been dreading this Saturday. It's the day Mark and I have agreed to review the bills piled on my desk.

When I was well, I was the money manager in our household, but lately I've shirked my duties. Mark has done his best to pick up the slack in this area, as he has everywhere else. I haven't had my ad agency job for going on two years now and, though I can keep my health benefits for three years, that still leaves me with astronomical out-of-pocket expenses for all my ER visits, hospital stays, and alternative healthcare. I haven't peeked at our online banking account in three months. I'm too scared to see the numbers in black and white.

But today, I've committed to face the music. We settle in to my office and log on to our accounts. First, we balance the checkbook together. After paying rent and utilities, due in three days, we have $319.23 in our checking account. Then I take the plunge and pull up our savings account. It's dwindled to about $1,000, from more than $13,000 just four months earlier.

Aghast, I turn to my husband. "Mark, what the hell happened to our savings account? There's nothing left."

"I kept having to transfer money into checking to cover

bills every month. And the move to L.A. wiped out a big chunk of it."

"Why didn't you tell me we were running out of money?" I say, my voice rising. "I knew things were bad, but I had no idea things were *this* bad!"

"I didn't tell you because I knew you would freak out, just like you're doing now!" Mark shoots back. "Besides, you told me NOT to talk to you about money so I haven't brought it up. I've been doing the best I can taking care of everything around here by myself. You can't scream at me for doing what you asked me to do."

He shifts uneasily in his seat. I'm still fuming, but I know he's right. There's nothing Mark could have done differently to improve our situation. I'm not making money. And Mark is busy rebuilding his career from scratch in this new city. Our primary source of income right now is my monthly disability check, which doesn't even cover our basic expenses. Even when I was feeling better and could supplement the disability income with consulting work, we were barely squeaking by. Naturally, we've fallen behind.

"Okay. Calm down," says Mark. He doesn't like having to talk about this any more than I do. "I have ten grand due to me in the next 90 days. And didn't you get a call about some consulting work a week ago?"

"That project won't even start for two months. The work will take a month and then it will be another month before I get paid. We don't even have enough to cover the rest of the things we need to pay *this* month. Even making the minimum payments on the credit card bills comes to more than $600."

We owe $15,573 to credit cards and $1,500 on our car loan. Just two years ago—back when I was making a six-figure income—we'd managed to pay off all our credit cards.

"We're going to have to use credit cards for gas and food this month. Who knows how we'll begin to put a dent in these medical bills?" I say, as I knock the pile of hospital bills onto the floor. Another $7,000 we don't have.

Mark looks like he wants to run out of the room, but I'm just getting started.

"Plus, we're still waiting to hear from the accountant about income taxes. The accountant's bill will be almost $2,000 even if we *don't* owe the IRS. And I'm going to need about $700 worth of dental work done soon."

I'm getting worked up. I feel angry, desperate, resentful, and overwhelmed all at once.

I start to sob. "Honey, we're screwed," I whimper.

Mark takes a deep breath and begins to rub his temples. "No, we're not," he says, taking on the role of the fixer now that I've crumpled. "We're just in debt. We'll figure out a way to work it out. You're just freaking out because you don't remember what it feels like to be in debt. You made shitloads of money for years and never had to worry about how to pay the bills. You just need to put things into perspective."

Well, he's right about my not having had to worry about money in the old days. But he's minimizing the problem with his usual habit of putting a good face on things. "Oh, they're in perspective, all right," I shoot back. "We're $30,000 in debt and can barely even cover our rent and utilities. I can't believe this is happening to us!" I'm close to shouting now.

"I'm not willing to sit here and talk about this anymore until you calm down," Mark says in his restrained, I'm-reminding-myself-that-I-love-you voice. He's much better at keeping his emotions in check than I am.

"Shit!" I scream and slam my fist on the desk three times, hard.

"Cami. Seriously. I'm going to leave the room. Come find me when you simmer down and can talk rationally." He calmly walks out of the room, which just pisses me off even more.

"How can you act so calm when we're *screwed?*" I yell after him. I see him shaking his head at me as he shuts the office door.

I move onto the couch in my office and throw a fit, pounding my fists on the cushions and screaming more cuss words. In the midst of my temper tantrum a series of thoughts bubble to the surface. *I'm not going to give anything to anyone anymore! I can't believe I was so stupid to think that giving away some spare change or a pair of old jeans could possibly help fix all the shit that's wrong in my life. I'm such an idiot!*

After pitching my fit alone, I decide I want an audience, so I call my mom.

Before I can launch into my story, Mom says, "So I decided I'm going to do your 29 days of giving." I had talked to her about my idea for the Giving Challenge during a phone call a few days ago. "I'm starting on April first and I'm going to try and get some friends to do it with me."

I can't bring myself to sound enthusiastic. "That's nice," I say to Mom.

"Don't sound so excited."

I immediately start to blubber out my tale of our debt and how Mark is an ass because he doesn't think it's a problem. After I wind down a little, my mom tells me she agrees with Mark.

"Honey, being $30,000 in debt really isn't the end of the world. All you have to do is work out a payment system with each creditor. You'll be able to start working part-time again soon and things will pick up for Mark now that you're in L.A. Don't do this to yourself. *It's only money.* What's important is that you start feeling better. And you know that Dad and I will help you guys out if you really need it."

"I can't believe I'm 35 years old and have to call daddy for a loan. How humiliating."

"Asking for help isn't humiliating, but it is humbling. And I know that's hard for you."

"Gee. Thanks, mom."

"I'm just telling you the truth. You've always been such a perfectionist. And you're so darn stubborn about doing everything yourself. There's no shame in letting others help you. Let me get Dad on the phone and we can all talk about this."

Hearing some soft mumbling on the other end of the phone, I stop crying and switch gears to talk to Dad.

"Hello," says my Dad from an extension.

"Hi Dad," I say. "How are you? I'm not having such a good day. I was just telling Mom that . . . that I'm having some money trouble." I can't believe how hard it is to say this. I made more money in my old job than he does. After a brief pause, I close my eyes and blurt it out: "I think I need to ask you guys for a loan." My face is burning.

"How much do you need?" My father always gets right to the point.

"Honestly?"

"Honestly."

I had only called to get my mother's sympathy. Now I was going to have to come up with a figure. Pushing past a sense of raw humiliation, I try to calculate what Mark and I might need to cover the bills until both of us start bringing in a little more money.

"Twenty thousand would be ideal. That would allow us to pay off most of our debt, except the one credit card that's on a zero percent introductory rate."

"That's a lot of money," Dad replies.

I'm desperate for his help, but he's not making it any easier. I'm seven years old again, hoping for a new bicycle. I'm 23 again, my business gone belly-up.

"I know," I tell him. "And if you can't do it, I totally understand. We could get credit counseling." I know this would ruin our chances of buying a house in the next few years, but I'd do it if we had to.

"No. I don't want you to ruin your credit again." He offers to lend us $16,000, to be paid back at very low interest on a schedule we can make work.

"We could afford to pay you back $300 a month starting in a little while. That would dramatically improve our situation." I'm just counting on Mark's business bringing in some steady money and mine getting going again.

"I can cut you a check later this week. I'll need a few days to set everything up through the bank." Dad is all business, which I appreciate at this moment.

I close my eyes, knowing how lucky I am to have someone to turn to when the well runs dry.

"Dad, I seriously don't know how to thank you for this," I say, feeling a sense of tremendous relief. My father and I had a harrowing time of it when I was a teenager, but I've always known I could count on him.

"I'm just glad we're in the position to help. Your mom and I had to get help from our parents a few times when we were starting out. Your Grandpa had to cosign the loan on our first house and help with the down payment."

When the conversation's over, I am grateful to be free of the panic that consumed me when I made the call. I find Mark in the living room watching TV and sit down next to him.

"Can we talk?" I ask him quietly.

He hits pause on the Tivo. "Sure. You seem calmer. Thank God."

"Well, I'm calmer because I called my parents and they just agreed to give us a $16,000 loan."

"What?" he explodes. "I can't believe you did that without talking to me first!" He jumps up, pacing in front of the forgotten TV.

"Mark, we need help." Now I'm the calm one while it's his turn to freak out.

"I'm mortified!" Mark says. "Your parents are going to think you married some freeloading jerk who can't take care of you."

And I thought *I* had a sensitive ego.

"They don't think that. They know we're in a bad situation because of my health and they want to help because they can."

I stand up and walk over to him, but he won't stop pacing.

"We are NOT taking their money," he barks.

"We're not *taking* the money; they're lending it to us. We're going to pay it back. With interest." I expect this to make him feel better.

He stops and turns to face me. "I can't believe this. What were you thinking? You should have come and talked to me about this before you called and asked for a loan. You didn't give us a chance to figure it out on our own. You just went running to mommy and daddy." He turns in disgust and resumes his angry pacing.

"Honey, I didn't mean to do it without consulting you. I just called my mom because I was panicking, and before I knew it, I was talking dollars and cents with my dad."

"Call them back and tell them we're not taking the loan. We can get a loan from our bank and consolidate all the debt."

"No. I'm not going to do that. We need the help. We'll be paying my dad a fraction of the interest rate we'd get at a bank. We're accepting the loan. Period."

"I hate it when you talk to me that way . . . like my opinions don't matter and you're the one who gets to make all the decisions for us."

"Well, I hate it when you act like an ego-driven idiot who can't admit when he needs help!"

We are both pissed now. And I know it's futile to keep talking.

"I'm going for my walk," I say. "Do you want to come with me?"

"No," says Mark. I can almost see the smoke spewing out of his ears.

I gather myself and my cane and hit the street for my daily laps. Maybe it's the adrenaline from all the emotion today, but I notice after two laps that I'm feeling pretty strong and steady on my feet. I decide to break the routine of only going around the block and head down Sunset Boulevard to a grocery store two blocks away.

When I reach the store, my face is flushed, so I sit on a bench to rest and then go inside to cool off in the air conditioning. I'm proud of myself for making the walk. I know that I can smooth things over with Mark and that this loan will take a lot of the stress out of our everyday lives. As I stand in the flower department smelling the roses, I begin to reflect on all the good things that have happened in the past ten days since I started the giving experiment.

I've begun booking consulting work again.

I got a free breakfast.

I've started walking every day.

I've been sleeping better.

I have been able to humbly accept my parents' help.

I don't want to stop these daily gifts, I think. *I'm going to see the 29 Days through.*

I'm thirsty, but I didn't bring my purse. Reaching into my jeans pocket for change, I am surprised to find a wadded up $20 bill that looks like it has gone through the wash. I walk over to the coffee counter and treat myself to a small iced tea.

I sit down to drink it and admire the flowers again. Roses

and white lilies are both on sale. I have just enough to get one bunch of each. Buying flowers always cheers me up, so on my way out, I purchase the blooms and then tuck them under my free arm as I leave the store, cane in hand.

Out in the parking lot an older woman is struggling to put her groceries into her trunk. She has permed silver hair and is wearing a lime green sheer scarf over her head. I reach her just as she loads the last bag, shuts the trunk and stops to wipe her brow. As she leans against the back of her car to rest, I stop right next to her. She smiles politely. I smile in return.

"Would you like some flowers?" I ask, separating off a few yellow roses and offering them to her.

"How much are they?" she asks.

"They're free. A gift."

She breaks into a huge grin and says, "Wonderful. Thank you," and reaches for the stems.

I'm instantly buoyed. On the walk home, I notice a red-headed woman walking a little black and white dog along the sidewalk across the street from my apartment building. I pull out some lilies from the bunch and cross the street to meet her as she reaches the corner.

"Would you like some flowers?" I ask.

"No, no. Is okay," she says in a heavy Russian accent.

She backs several steps away from me, as if I am someone to fear.

I step toward her slowly and hold out the lilies.

"Are you sure? They smell really good," I say as I take a big whiff and then extend an open bloom toward her.

She sniffs in its scent and her face opens into a smile.

"Oh goodness. Yummy," she says and giggles like a little girl.

"Please take them. They're a gift. For you," I say.

She takes the stems from me with a "Thanks," and heads across the street.

"When you practice mindful connections with others," I can hear Mbali saying, "your life *feels* meaningful and so it is."

I amble slowly up the steps and find Mark on the couch where I left him an hour earlier, now watching an episode of *60 Minutes*. I put the remaining flowers in a vase with some water and then join him on the couch. He pauses the Tivo again.

"I'm sorry," I say. "I should have talked to you before accepting the money from my parents."

"I'm sorry, too," he says. "I know we need the help."

He takes a breath. "It's hard for me to imagine going to *my* family for money—no one would be able to lend us anything. But I know if my Dad was alive or my Mom was in a position to help, they wouldn't hesitate. And I probably wouldn't feel weird about taking a loan from her. I just have to accept that it's okay to ask for help right now."

I'm so relieved Mark's not still angry with me.

"I'm tired," I say. "I just walked all the way to the grocery store and back."

"Wow. That's great, hon. I'm so glad you're feeling stronger."

Mark extends his open arms to me, and I settle in beside him with my head on his chest. I can hear his heart beating. I sit up to adjust the vase of flowers on the coffee table in front of us and smile, knowing that two other women in L.A. have the same flowers in their house this evening. Then I rest my head back on Mark's shoulder. Breathing in tandem with Mark, I feel a sense of serenity that has eluded me for most of the day.

gift 12 ~ Birthday Poem

SUNDAY, MARCH 30

I've developed an addiction to Post-It notes over the past two years, since the MS started making it hard for me to remember things. If my stash runs low, I get nervous.

I often pilfer several pads at a time from Mark's office and hoard them in my desk drawers, which drives him crazy because he can never find his own Post-Its when he needs them. At least once a week he comes stomping into my office and yanks open my top desk drawer exclaiming, "Why are you always stealing my Post-Its? If you need more, just tell me, and I'll get you some. Sheesh!"

I've never explained my need for these colorful little sticky pieces of paper because that would mean admitting that my brainpower isn't what it used to be. Mark already knows this, of course. He's constantly trailing along behind me, turning off stove burners and shutting the refrigerator door. "Can't you pay more attention to things, Cami?" he pleads with me ten times a day.

I can't bring myself to tell him that I *am* paying attention, but that it doesn't seem to make any difference. I still forget things all the time. I put soup on to heat and forget it's there until all the liquid has boiled off and the house starts to stink of charred lentils. About three months ago, I stopped trying to cook altogether for fear of burning the house down. That wasn't too hard to give up. But a lot of my self-identity hinges on being "intelligent." And intelligent people don't forget things all the time. So I obsessively write things down on Post-Its—things I need to remember from day to day, random notes and ideas—and stick them all over my walls and desk. About once a month I collect them all and organize them into the appropriate sections in my notebooks.

I have one book devoted to my business. My business card is taped to the outside cover, and inside are sections designated for different clients, marketing ideas, business development plans, and partnership possibilities. Another notebook labeled "Health" is full of notes on things people have mentioned to me, plus articles and web printouts about health items I might want to look into in the future. A third book with a purple cover is dedicated to creative writing. This isn't organized at all. It's just crammed full of Post-Its with story ideas, lines of poetry, and scribbled notes about significant experiences I want to write about someday.

I never identify myself as a "writer," but I've been writing since I was a kid. I submitted my first article to a magazine when I was 11 years old. Three half-baked novels sit on my hard drive, plus lots of short stories, personal essays, and over one million words of material for memoirs. I haven't touched any of those pages in more than two years. Before I got sick, I had a blog that attracted a lot of traffic and even won some awards. I bared my soul on that site and told highly personal stories about my life and my struggles with mental illness, addiction, and food issues. People often took time to write to me themselves, disclosing painful and intimate details from their lives. My sad tales helped compel many people (including myself, eventually) to seek help.

Like everything else I wrote, that blog came from the drama and trauma of my past. But when I met Mark, I wanted to stop defining myself by my "mental illness," so I took down the blog and didn't produce anything for a long time. I didn't want to write again until I could do it in a new voice, one not born of illness. For the longest time, I couldn't even comply with a simple request from Mbali to put in writing the things I needed help letting go of along with something new to take their place. Finally I managed to write that I wanted to let go of illness and replace it with health.

I reach onto the top shelf of my desk and pull out an empty little lime green notebook. I take out a blue Sharpie and write "29 Gifts" on the cover. Next I slowly stick all of my gift-related Post-Its inside in chronological order. I jot down a few additional ideas and transfer all the notes I've written into my day planner for each day I've given something. Now there's a place for me to capture the important things I'll want to remember later.

I turn on my computer and start to make files for my gift-giving and for the wider giving movement. I'm having fun surfing the web when pain suddenly shoots down my neck into my back. *Damn it,* I think. *I used to get lost in web research or writing, working for long blissful spells. Lately, I'm lucky if I can last an hour at the keyboard.*

Then a more positive voice inside my head tells me, *Be grateful for the hour, then. At least your hands worked well enough to type today.* I'm pleased to hear this voice. It's been a while since she's piped up.

I am feeling the giving spirit today. My commitment to the Challenge bloomed again yesterday when I handed out the flowers to those two women on the street. The look of pleasure that washed over the Russian woman's face when she smelled that lily sent a happy rush of energy through my body. I want to feel more of that. I was so moved by making a meaningful connection with a stranger.

Mark's not up yet, so I prepare a little gift for Jeff. I'll see him at church later and can give it to him there.

I sit down on the floor and pull a gold box off my bottom bookshelf. Inside are some rocks I collected last time I was able to go on a real hike, which was when I was still living in San Francisco. I take out one of the gray and white rocks and recall what it felt like to walk along the Lands End trail that day, the soaring cliffs above and Pacific Ocean crashing on the rocks below. It's always chilly near the water in the Bay Area so I was bundled into a scarf and windbreaker. On my walk back to the car, I picked up some rocks that I thought were unique or pretty and filled my two deep pockets until they were bulging and sagging under the stony weight. I've always loved the notion that a weighty object can help keep something of importance top of mind, so I gave them away to friends as "gratitude rocks" over the next year whenever I felt moved to do so. Now I have only three left.

I select one for Jeff and rub a little essential oil onto its surface. I drop the rock into a small cellophane bag and tie it shut with an orange ribbon. On the outside of the bag I stick one of the labels I've made up to go with the rocks:

Your Gratitude Rock

Consciously practicing gratitude is the most powerful way to attract more abundance in your life. Hold this rock during your daily meditation, put it where you'll see it each day, or carry it in your pocket as a reminder to reflect on the things you're grateful for. This will help you attract more of what you want into your life.

I picked this rock for you from the Coastal Trail Beach and I have charged it with love and appreciation for you. It has been treated with essential oils of lavender, white sage and grapefruit.

With love and gratitude ~ Cami

I take a box of greeting cards off the shelf. My mother makes cards out of scrapbooking materials, which is kind of funny since she and Dad own a pharmacy filled with aisles of cards. But she likes making cards so much that she has way more than she can use and regularly sends little piles to me.

I find a bright red card that says FRIENDS on the front and sit down to write a note to Jeff to thank him for committing to the 29 Gifts. Then I package everything into a little gift bag that I happen to have on hand. Along with a love of crafts, keeping stashes of gift bags and wrapping paper in the house is another of my mother's habits that I inherited.

When we arrive at church, I see Jeff in the parking lot. We wave at each other and he comes over to say hi.

"I brought you a little gift," I say with a smile.

"I love this game." He laughs and takes the package.

After church, Mark and I sit and talk with Jeff.

"Since I started giving a week ago, I booked a gig working

on a video game that will last at least a month," he tells us, "and a few other possibilities seem to have popped up out of nowhere!"

I'm so pleased. "So, do you think the giving has helped turn things around?" I ask him.

"I really do. It's like I'm expecting good things to happen now," he says.

I know what he means. Though I still have my bad moments, I'm more ready to believe in at least the possibility that good things might come my way. I might even miss giving gifts when the 29 Days are up.

Back at home, I lie down for an hour to rest. Later we'll be driving to our friend Lydia's for a birthday party in honor of her brother, Nick. But first I squeeze in five laps around the block. I'm feeling steady on my feet, so I try it without my cane today. For the past week I've been practicing walking up and down our long hallway without the cane. It's relatively safe because there are walls within arm's distance that I can reach to steady myself. Mark comes with me and we celebrate my solo flight: My steps are slow and careful as I circle the block, but we're thrilled that I take them completely on my own.

High on the success, we pack ourselves into the car for Nick's party. We hang around chatting and devouring great Mexican food, which Lydia's boyfriend prepared. The small group settles into the living room to blow out candles and eat chocolate cake, then the real ceremony begins.

Nick, a poetry lover, had requested that everyone bring some creative writing to read aloud. All the family members read funny, creative odes celebrating Nick. Two of his cousins even get up and perform their poem, complete with music and dance. Lydia reads a couple of limericks that family members who live in other states e-mailed especially for the event. By the time it's my turn to read, I'm feeling embarrassed because I didn't understand that we were expected to write something expressly for Nick. In fact, my piece seems more inappropriate by the minute. Everyone is looking at me and my sheet of paper expectantly.

Crap, I fret. *Maybe I can play the I-don't-feel-well card to get out of reading my piece. They'll let me off the hook.* But then I tell myself, *You should go ahead and read this. It's your gift to Nick, even if it's not about him.* It's a kind of ecological ode I wrote while sitting by the Russian River in Northern California.

"I'm sorry," I say to the birthday boy and everyone else in the room. "I'm not really a poet. I just brought a piece of prose that I wrote a long time ago."

"That's great," says Nick. "Let's hear it!"

I feel my heart begin to pound and my throat close. I hate reading out loud in front of people, especially my own work. I take a deep breath. Then I begin to read, my voice trembling at first, then with more ease. By the time I'm halfway through, I've forgotten that the piece doesn't directly fit the day:

I lean back on my elbows and close my eyes to ponder what this river knows about each of us. I bet it can testify to more of our lives than we'd believe possible. I'll bet it remembers the aqua blue headband you wore the day you met your husband on the bridge upstream. It could probably tell you the secret ingredients in your grandma's tart apple pie that she used to bring to the family picnics by the big oak tree on the north shore. I bet the river even knows that you used to steal packs of Bazooka bubble gum from the corner store if the cashier wasn't looking when you went with your dad on a quick beer or cigarette run—you in your yellow-and-black polka-dot swimsuit with the ruffle across the butt and river sand between your bare toes.

As I doze on the riverbank and let the flowing water ease my sadness, I think to myself what a perfect companion it really is to us all. It listens, but doesn't judge. It understands, but doesn't preach. It embraces us in familiar acceptance and reminds us that when we've all gone back to the earth and the light that made everything out of nothing, it will still be here. Flowing. Singing our song.

The room is silent for a few seconds after I finish.

"Wow. That was wonderful," says Nick.

"I didn't realize you're such a good writer. I thought you were a business consultant or something," says Lydia.

"I am. But I'm a writer, too." The word echoes in my head. I've never identified myself that way out loud before. I turn to Nick and smile, "Happy Birthday. Thank you for letting me join in the fun."

I feel a surge of possibility and recall one of Mbali's precepts: *The best way to attract abundance into your life is to be in a perpetual state of giving and gratitude.* I may have hoped for better health, but I don't think I dared until this moment to think I could truly embrace myself as a writer.

gift 13 ~ Meter Maid

"Mark!" I poke my head into Mark's office and interrupt him recording an audition for a car commercial to tell him my good news. "I just booked consulting sessions with four new clients! And a fifth one wants to buy an eight-hour package!"

This means I'll have $2,700 worth of business booked for April, plus the $3,000 gig that will start the following month. All I'd done was update my website and make it clear I was open for business. I didn't expect much work to come my way for a while. I feel a sense of relief that we'll be able to start paying my dad's loan back right away.

"Congratulations, hon!" Mark says and gives me a squeeze. "We should celebrate! Let's go out for breakfast."

I start to leave without my cane, but Mark objects.

"The café is several blocks away," he says. "If you can't walk back, I don't want to have to carry you that far. Don't get all cocky and start heading too far from home without the cane."

My practical husband. I grudgingly agree and come back to pick up the cane.

In the restaurant, Mark drowns his pancakes in butter and syrup while I enjoy a plate of scrambled eggs with spinach. Our conversation drifts to when we might want to try to get pregnant.

After we got engaged, we started trying to conceive right away because we didn't want to wait to have kids. We tried even harder for the first year after I got sick, then we had to stop when I agreed to go on the immunosuppressant injections the doctors insisted upon. I'd have to go off this medication—something we've agreed is not worth the risk right now—to try again. That's just one complication. No matter how much we want a baby, we've been grappling with whether that would become another huge responsibility to fall squarely on Mark's shoulders.

This is not the time to hash all that out. It just feels good to be having a conversation that doesn't erupt into an argument.

We walk home holding hands. Our friends Megan and JJ from San Francisco are stopping by later, so I nap for two hours and then get up to shower and dress.

Mark answers the door when Megan and JJ ring and we give them a tour of our apartment. Megan and JJ comment on how large the space is and how "San Francisco–like" it feels.

"That's why we decided to take the place," Mark says. "After living in San Francisco so long, this place felt like home." Soon JJ and Mark are deep into a discussion about music. As they debate the merits of old Bon Jovi and the Beatles, Megan and I catch up. She is a client as well as a friend, so we talk about her business.

"You know, Cami, it's going so well," she says contentedly. "I just signed a lease for a new office space."

After a while it's time for Mark to leave for his auditions. Megan, JJ, and I follow him out the door for a late lunch.

Megan has to drive around for awhile before finding a parking spot. Instinctively, I dig five quarters out of my purse and plug the meter.

"It's my gift for the day," I tell Megan. She's one of the people I had e-mailed about the 29 Gifts.

We go to Urth Café on Melrose and chat, then head over to the Bohdi Tree, a metaphysical bookstore Megan knows about. I love the place, with its spiritual literature and trinkets. Megan and I are both suckers for anything we jokingly refer to as "woo-woo," so we have fun pointing things out to each other. I spend a lot of time in the used book section and end up buying *The Courage to Give*. I like the title, so I buy it without even reading the back cover.

I'm feeling kind of tired after being out for a couple of hours, and Megan and JJ need to get to the airport to catch their flight home. They drive me back to my apartment and we hug our goodbyes. As soon as the door closes, someone knocks. It's Megan.

"I almost forgot to give you this," she says. She's holding out a check for $300, part of an outstanding balance she's owed me for months. She's been paying me whenever she can.

"Thanks!" I say. "I could really use this right now."

She smiles. "Glad I could help then." We hug goodbye one more time, and she runs back to the car.

After I settle in on the couch, I start reading *The Courage to Give* and get another surprise. The author, Jackie Waldman, is a woman with MS who found relief through giving. She has published a whole series of books on different topics. Each book is a collection of thirty essays about people who have found creative ways to give back to their communities.

I start thinking about my giving project again. Soon I'll see what Eve has dreamed up for the website design. It's fun to have my friends involved. I indulge myself in dreaming of the possibilities that could lie ahead for me.

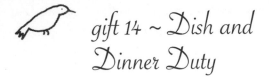

gift 14 ~ Dish and Dinner Duty

TUESDAY, APRIL 1

When I began working with Mbali, she suggested I build altars in my home—places of devotion where I could make offerings to my ancestors and to the great spirit that unites us all. Now I have little altars all over my house. I pause in front of one I recently made on a bookshelf. On one shelf is a photo of my grandmother and both of my grandfathers, all of whom died during my twenties. There is no photo of my living grandmother because Mbali stresses that it's important not to put images of people who are still alive on ancestral altars. I've also lined up two teddy bears that were hand sewn from pieces of old clothing from all four of my grandparents, several shells and rocks I've collected over the years, a statue of Shiva—the Hindu god of transformation—a large piece of rose quartz I was given by a reiki master years ago in Nebraska, and a porcupine quill that Mbali gave me during my first divination.

I pick up the large brown-and-white striped quill and smile as I recall that day over a year ago when I sat across from Mbali on the floor of her Oakland living room. Between us was spread her cloth with symbols painted on it, and in its center lay a small pile of rocks, shells, and bones. The divination begins with a question posed to your ancestors, something you've been struggling with that they might help you answer. Mbali uses cowrie shells, the shells of sea snails, which have a glossy finish and a narrow opening, like a slit, on the underside.

"What is your question today?" Mbali asked me as I adjusted myself into a cross-legged position to get more comfortable.

"I have been feeling stuck creatively for some time now. I feel like this lack of creative outlet is related to my illness."

"Okay. So what is the question?"

"I'm not sure. I want to know how I can get myself to start writing again."

Mbali smiled at me and a little knowing laugh escaped her plump lips. Articulating the question you want guidance about during a divination is usually a struggle. "So your question is how can you begin writing again? Remember, it's good to be specific."

"No. It's not just that. For years I wrote from a place of pain. I used to publish my work online and had a big audience that followed my stories. I mainly wrote about some horrors in my past and the later struggles I had with depression, addiction, and eating disorders." Saying all this out loud helped me define it and focus on what I wanted to work through that day.

"Writing was like therapy for me back then," I continued. "After years of this type of writing, plus a lot of counseling and addiction treatment, I found myself well and happy, which was great. But I didn't know how to write from this healthier place, so I just stopped. I felt like I lost my voice. I just didn't have anything to say."

"Hmmm. We're getting closer," said Mbali, her brown eyes locking onto my baby blues. "So you want to know how you can find a new writing voice?"

"Yes. How can I find a new writing voice that communicates from a place of love, hope, and faith?"

"There we go. That's a good, specific question. So why do you want this?" she asked gently.

I hesitated. I couldn't find an answer. After a long pause, Mbali asked, "Are you done with the pain?"

Bingo. I hadn't been able to word it that way to myself. "Yes," I nodded. "I want to move past it but still hold on to the creative instincts that make me want to write."

"All right. Now state your question as you spread the minerals out on the cloth."

I reached into the pile in front of her and began to move my hand through it in a circular pattern. After a few seconds, the question resonated in the room—*How can I find a new writing voice that communicates from love, hope, and faith?*

Mbali pointed to a red stone that had settled itself between a small piece of bone and a shimmery pink crystal.

"Who is this?" she asked and threw her three cowrie shells next to her right foot. "This red stone represents one of your male ancestors who is here to provide guidance. Do you know who he is?"

"It might be my grandpa—my mother's father, William," I guessed.

Mbali threw her shells again. "No. The shells say it's not William."

"Hmm. Maybe my dad's father, my grandpa Floyd."

The shells hit the cloth between us again, and Mbali n[o]ded her head yes. "It's Floyd," she confirmed.

Mbali told me she was getting a message that it was time for me to come home to my body because it was safe now. "You cannot write from a disembodied state," she told me.

"I don't really understand what you mean," I replied, perplexed.

"You're lacking connection with yourself right now. You're not allowing yourself to feel your emotions or process your fears. You're denying yourself. Your creative expression is rooted in your relationship with yourself, which needs to be cultivated right now."

This rang true for me. "Floyd, my grandpa, was a farmer; he knew how to cultivate things and make them grow," I told her.

Mbali proposed that I go out into nature and plant some seeds to symbolically fuel my creativity. "Ask the earth to help you grow a new voice," she suggested with wisdom and compassion.

Mbali also told me that Mark and I would be moving to a new home soon in Southern California. She warned that I wasn't going to be happy about the move but that I needed to embrace it because I wasn't settled in my true home yet. At the time, I thought this was crazy because I had no intention of moving south, yet here I am standing in my new house in Los Angeles. The porcupine quill I am holding right now fell out of Mbali's head wrap three times during the divination. Each time it fell, she would pick it up and stick it back in the folds of blue fabric that protected her head. The fourth time the quill fell out, she picked it up and handed it to me.

"The ancestors are clearly telling me to give this to you. Treat it with care. It was given to me by one of my teachers and it is very special."

I took the smooth quill from her and nodded my thanks.

We covered a lot of territory in that session, which sprang from one specific question but traveled out to encompass my thoughts about my parents, my illness, and some difficult scenes from my youth. Part intuitive, part life coach, Mbali sent me on my way with hope that I could carve a path for myself away from this "stuck" place.

On my way home I stopped at a garden shop to pick up some sunflower seeds, which I planted into a patch of dirt near my apartment building. While I patted down the earth on top of them, I sent out a silent plea to the universe: *Please help me find a new writing voice that communicates from love, hope, and faith.*

Then I got into bed and slept for thirteen straight hours. When I awoke, I cracked open a journal and wrote the first story I'd written in nearly two years. Not surprisingly, it was about my grandfather.

That first divination pulled the plug out of my jug, and I filled two journals over the next nine months while I took part in a monthly healing circle that Mbali led. All the women in the group were drawn to our circle by a common call. During those meetings, we laughed and cried and sang and danced together. We meditated and made masks, medicine bags, and talismans. We did rituals out in nature and spoke our true desires and deepest fears to one another.

Many of us began to make significant changes in our lives. One woman left her job to pursue her passions. One left an unhappy marriage. Another decided to set out on a solo trek through South America. I began to make peace with my diagnosis, to some extent, and started to accept the changes it was bringing to my life—like the move to Los Angeles—and I wrote and wrote and wrote. Stories and poems tumbled out of me, an avalanche of pent-up words.

And now here I stand just a few months later, poised for whatever may come next. I say my affirmation for today, "*Today I give with joy,*" and smile to myself.

I feel strong today, faster and less wobbly, so I do five laps around the block, sans cane. Even those steep stairs feel like less of a threat as I arrive back home.

I walk into the kitchen and attack the sink full of dishes. I rinse a stack of ceramic plates, humming to myself. This is a gift to Mark, who is gone today recording a commercial. I haven't helped out around our house for months. Now that I'm feeling stronger, it's time to pitch in where I can.

Soon all the dishes are drying in the rack. I sit down at my computer and write a summary of my gifts for the last few days, then I pull out my file for Allie, my friend and client who arrives tomorrow afternoon. I jot down a few ideas I want to share with her, then make a salad for dinner.

Mark is shocked to come home to food and a clean kitchen. "You really *must* be feeling better if you cooked!" he jokes. We sit down in our dining room to eat.

"Making salad isn't really cooking," I remind him.

"There's chicken in this salad. That's cooked."

"It was left over from something you cooked a couple of days ago."

"What about the beets in here? They're cooked, aren't they?"

"I boiled some water and threw them in. Technically they're cooked."

"Well, they're delicious!" Mark says.

"I wanted to do something nice for you. To say thank you for everything you've done."

"What do you mean?"

"God, Mark, everything! Cleaning and washing clothes and driving me to the doctor millions of times. I really appreciate you."

"I'm your husband," says Mark. "If the tables were turned, you'd be here for me."

"Honey, I'm not sure how I would have responded if you'd gotten sick. I don't know if I could have stepped up the way you have."

"You're a good person, Cami. You would have stepped up. Someday I'll need you to be here for me, and I know you will be."

Mark takes my hand and kisses the back of each finger. "Have I told you today that I love you?"

"No, actually," I tease him. "This is the first time we've seen each other today."

"Well, I do. I love you. Whether you boil beets or not. I love you, babe."

"I love you, too."

gift 15 ~ Cane and Able

I watch Allie clicking up my stairs in her designer heels and say a silent prayer of thanks that she's my first client as I start back to work. There couldn't be a better way to begin than with the woman I call Firecracker Allie. When she enters a room you can't help but notice. She's blond and busty—and brainy to boot.

"Sweet Cami, it's so great to see you," bursts Allie as she envelops me in a warm hug. Her hair tickles my face as I start to tear up. It's such a relief to see one of my San Francisco friends for the first time in several months.

Allie is getting ready to relaunch her consulting company for women entrepreneurs. Today we will be brainstorming ideas for her new venture. We decide to start our day with a working lunch at a nearby restaurant.

We both put on some sneakers. Remembering Mark's advice, I reach into the corner where I always keep my cane. It's not there. Little flutters of worry build in my stomach as I go in and out of every room in the house searching for it. I phone Mark, out on an audition, who says he hasn't seen the cane in two days, not since Monday morning when we went out for breakfast. I track back through the last couple of days and realize that Monday is the last day I used it. I know I took it to breakfast in the morning that day and am *pretty sure* I took it with me when Megan, JJ, and I went to lunch and the bookstore. I look up the phone numbers and call these places to ask if they have a brightly decorated cane that says, "*Not every adventure happens in a storybook*" on it. No luck.

"Holy shit!" I say to Allie, who has settled into one of my dining room chairs, a spectator to my frantic search. "I walked away from my cane sometime on Monday."

"Whooo hooo!" responds Allie.

"No. Not whooo hooo. I need it. Plus, I custom-made the thing. It was one-of-a-kind. It's so cool looking. I'll never be able to replicate it."

Allie has a baffled expression on her face. "Are you talking about a cane or a freaking Birkin bag? Girl, I think the fact that it's gone is a sign that you don't need it anymore. Look at you. You're walking great."

"Right now I am, but some days I still lurch around. I bet someone found it and stole it to give to their great aunt Ester."

"Yeah, because great aunt Ester needs a damn cane and you don't."

At that, an unwilling laugh escapes me.

"Maybe you're right," I sigh. "Let's just go. If I get weak, we can always stop at a pharmacy or grocery store to buy a cheap replacement."

"That's the spirit!" says Allie as she links arms with me to walk down the stairs and out the door.

"So what is it about L.A.?" she asks after we've walked three blocks down Sunset Boulevard. "Why is there a donut shop on every block, but everyone is a skinny bitch? Who the hell eats all the donuts?"

"Maybe they're all fronts to launder drug money."

We've known each other for two years, business colleagues who evolved into friends. When I ask for an update on the dating front, Allie tells me all about the guy she's being set up with next weekend. She digs her BlackBerry out of her bag to show me a photo of him.

"Isn't he hunky? He's six-three. And look, he even has all of his hair."

"He is pretty hunky. But you really shouldn't turn away balding guys. Mark's hair is thinning, but he's still hot."

"Believe me, having hair isn't a requirement on my list," says Allie as she tosses her BlackBerry back into her purse. "It's just a nice bonus."

We chat and laugh our way down the Walk of Fame to Hollywood Boulevard and Highland, ending up at a little pizza place.

"So what do you want to start with?" I ask Allie after our waiter has delivered the cheese pizza and chopped salad that we're splitting.

She pulls out a piece of paper and unfolds it: "This."

The paper is covered with little sketched symbols, split into four quadrants: little stick people, dollar signs, arrows, handshakes, and at least forty other drawings, like something my nine-year-old niece could have produced.

"What the hell is this?" I ask.

"It's my new marketing plan tool. These four quadrants represent the four primary advertising channels—in person, online, in print, or promotion. And each of the symbols represents a specific tactical method within the channel. This little icon is for e-mail. And the envelope is a direct mail package. The person with the talk bubble is a word-of-mouth referral."

She devours a cherry tomato as I move from confusion to admiration. "When I take a client through this," she goes on, "I ask them a series of questions to help them decide which channels they'll focus their marketing energy on, then help them home in on the tactics. I talk about everything in plain English, using really simple terms."

"It's brilliant!" I say.

"Thanks! I'm trying to come up with a new way to package my services and rebrand myself. I've been doing start-up consulting for a couple of years now and find that most of my clients need things to be super-simple. They don't get the marketing mumbo jumbo, so I'm going to stop speaking that language."

I also work with start-up companies, and Allie is absolutely right. Most entrepreneurs like to keep things simple. "You should call it the Stick Figure Marketing Plan," I suggest.

"Oh my God! That's perfect." Allie scrawls the name across the top of the page. "We can check that one off the list. Now let's go reinvent my entire business model."

We have a lively and productive lunch, and Allie picks up the tab. The whole way back to my house we comment on how different L.A. feels than San Francisco, pointing out every pair of designer shoes we see women teetering around on. Allie and I are both shoe junkies, though MS put a stop to my addiction to high heels. Put me in a pair of heels these days and I'll be on my ass in no time. Now I just have to live vicariously through girlfriends like Allie.

After my panic, I don't even miss the cane. In fact, I don't give it another thought during Allie's entire two-day visit.

We spend two more hours that afternoon brainstorming changes to Allie's business model and make so much progress that we decide to go for massages at Grace Healing Center around the corner from my house. I pay for her massage as my gift for the day.

We top off our evening by cooking dinner together—a curried lentil dish with rice that we whip up in less than thirty minutes. When Mark comes home to a warm plate of food, he nearly falls over in shock. I'm working, I'm doing some daily household tasks, and I'm still managing to walk every single day. The improvements in the last couple of weeks seem almost too good to be true.

Tomorrow Allie and I will finish our work, but the real priority will be to hit a few boutiques on Melrose. My task is to help her pick out a cute outfit for the blind date. It's a modest little plan, but I haven't enjoyed any simple pleasures in months. I may never be rid of the MS, but I can learn to keep it from preventing little outings like this.

gift 16 ~ Love Letter

Allie is working away on her laptop before I'm even awake. She's wearing a pair of tight stretchy pants most women over the age of 25 wouldn't dare to pick up in a store, let alone try on and purchase. Her pink, long-sleeved T-shirt is stretched equally tight. Her hair is in a ponytail on top of her head.

"Sorry girl, ya caught me before the bra went on," Allie chirps as I sit down in my comfy chair across from her perch on my baby blue couch. She slept on the couch in my home office and has already put it back together. The sheets are now folded neatly over the arm of the sofa. Paper is littered all over the cushions and the coffee table in front of her.

Allie pulls her arms out of both sleeves, flips her shirt up and puts on a black, lacy bra, talking all the while. "I decided to get to work on the brand platform worksheet you gave me. I think I've got some good ideas brewing."

I give the sort of little nervous laugh you offer up when someone points out your hot pink underwear is showing through your white skirt. I decide to ignore the peep show and respond with, "Holy crap. I knew you were an early bird, but it looks like you've been awake and working for hours. I'm barely functioning."

"Yeah. I woke up at five o'clock, so I figured, why wait?"

"That was two and a half hours ago!" I say. "You must be starving."

We clamor around the kitchen getting a quick breakfast and then shut ourselves into my office to work. In a matter of three short hours, we hammer out a new brand strategy for Allie's business and a number of good names and tagline ideas. Our favorite is *YES Network: You Equal Success*, but we're not sold on it and decide to let it stew for a few weeks. It will actually be several months before Allie and her partner will succeed in launching a new venture, Hatch Network, which offers education and resources for women entrepreneurs nationwide.

After we roll up our big pages of notes, I take Allie out for a celebratory coffee as my gift for the day.

"Let the shopping begin!" I declare as we leave the coffeehouse. It feels so good to be out doing something normal. I'll never take the fun of shopping with my girlfriends for granted again.

Allie pulls me into a little boutique called Mannequins. She wants to go in because she saw the store on an episode of *The Hills*. We're both addicted to reality shows. I watch as my boisterous friend tries on a number of outfits for her date, finally settling on a sexy little black dress and a very cool canary yellow shirt, which she says will look great with jeans. She's not sure what she and this guy will be doing so she wants both casual and dressy options. She pays for her purchase and then turns to look at me. Scanning my sad outfit, she declares, "Cami, those jeans are huge. Why the hell are you wearing them? They don't fit."

"I know. They're my only pair of jeans and I've dropped 20 pounds in the past few months. It's muscle waste."

"Gee. What a bummer," Allie says sarcastically. "Wish I could lose 20 pounds without even trying." If it were anyone but Allie, I'd be pretty pissed at such an insensitive comment. Instead I give her a wry smile.

"Believe me," I say to set her straight, "you don't want to go through what I've experienced. What I wouldn't give to have that 20 pounds back and just erase the last few months."

"Sorry. You're right," she says, cringing. "But we have to buy you some jeans that fit. The butt is so baggy it looks like you took a dump in your pants." Allie motions to the sales associate. They both tear into the racks and start pulling out pair after pair of jeans. They send me into a dressing room with a huge stack and insist I try them *all* on and model them. They pull a bunch of tops, too, because Allie says my boring green T-shirt just won't do.

Forty-five minutes later, I leave the store with two pairs of jeans and two shirts, all on sale. I put the total on my credit card. I know I'll get a check from Allie, but I already feel guilty about spending the money and I start to worry out loud.

"Stop whining, kiddo," Allie tells me. "Just think of this as your gift to yourself for the day." She knows about my giving experiment and has agreed to try it, too.

"I don't know if giving to myself counts," I say to her. "And, you know, it's our second anniversary today. I really should have bought a gift for Mark."

"Of course giving to yourself counts!" exclaims Allie. "If

you aren't being nice to yourself, you won't have the energy to be nice to other people."

She has a good point, so I decide to embrace my new clothes as a gift. We hit a few men's stores on our way back down Melrose, but I don't find anything I think Mark will like. He's really picky about clothes, so I'm afraid to choose anything for him.

Though I've tried several times, I still haven't managed to convince Mark to try the Giving Challenge and sign up to share stories. He thinks it's uncool to "brag" about the things you do for others. I've told him that the reason I write stories about my gifts is to inspire more people to give, not to brag. Plus, it allows us to share gift ideas with each other. He says he'll think about it, but I'm not sure he'll come around.

Allie drives me back to my house and rushes off to catch her flight home. It was so wonderful spending time with my sparkplug of a friend and getting some good work done.

I go upstairs and make a nice card for Mark, using some photos of us to make a collage. Then I write him a gooey love letter. He loves that stuff. Luckily, I happen upon an iTunes gift card in my desk that I'd forgotten about, sent to me by a client a while ago. He is a huge music lover, so I'm glad he'll have something to open on this special day.

Mark and I exchange our gifts over take-out Chinese at home that evening and toast the positive changes we're seeing with sparkling cider. I think back to the day he proposed. He came into the dining room after cooking us a wonderful breakfast—I was still wearing my old flannel pajamas. He made a big production out of lifting a lid off a plate to reveal . . . nothing.

"Oh shit," he said. "I can't believe I screwed this up." He reached into his back pocket and fumbled nervously, dropping the plate on the floor and breaking it.

"I forgot to put it on the plate. I'm so nervous," he said sheepishly, pulling a little ring box out from behind his back. He got down onto one knee and then took out a love letter, which he began to read to me, and then he asked me to be his wife. I was in tears by the third word of the letter, and after his proposal I threw my arms around him, crying like a baby.

On this second anniversary, we reminisce about the early days of our courtship and we each reread the love letters we wrote to each other the night before we got married. I'm reminded once again how lucky I am to have found the man I want to share my life with.

gift 17 ~ $100 I'd Like to Keep

"Giving of any kind begins the process of change and moves us to remember that we are part of a much greater universe," Mbali had explained to me. I recall something else that I haven't wanted to think about in a while. "What if," she proposed, "you were to give away something you felt you could never part with?"

Yesterday's shopping spree notwithstanding, money is the thing I have the most trouble parting with. I should know better. I've always received the money I need to take care of myself, but I still fall into "scarcity thinking" sometimes . . . especially lately, as a new stack of bills arrives on our doorstep each month to add to the looming pile. Mbali says you will rarely move back into a place of scarcity when you remember to give mindfully each day.

So today I decide to dig deep. What can't I part with right now? How about a hundred bucks?

I've committed to this sum—a nice round number high enough to feel like a stretch—even though I honestly don't feel we have the money to spare. No question that $100 could be put to good use chipping away at those bills. Even though I got a check from Allie for our work together, a five-figure debt still looms over us. And though most of it is owed to my father now instead of credit card companies and health care providers, I still feel a pressing urge to pay the loan back as quickly as possible.

I take a deep breath and write out a check to support Eve's South Africa teaching mission. Helping her with her fundraising letter the other day really showed me how great the need for education is in that country. Eve will be working with adolescents to teach them technology skills, in addition to mentoring on other topics. It feels really good signing the check and popping it in the mail. I make the check out directly to Eve instead of to Worldteach, the nonprofit organization that is sponsoring her trip. This way I can't claim a tax deduction. Somehow the gift seems more "pure" that way.

When I log on to the 29 Gifts website to write about today's gift in my blog, I'm surprised to see that Mark has posted a giving story. He must have come home from auditions and tiptoed into his office to write it up. I read his account of Gift 1 with a little tingle of pleasure that he's finally on board:

> Last week, I was talking with this girl at a casting company and the topic of Paul McCartney came up because I had just met his touring guitar player, Brian Ray, in Santa Monica moments before. It was kind of a big deal for me being a McCartney/Beatles freak and all. She went on to tell me that having seen McCartney during his '89 tour was one of the best shows she'd ever seen. In the back of my mind, I made a mental note of that.
>
> I knew I had to go back into that casting office today, so knowing this girl's affinity for McCartney, I quickly whipped up a CD mix called "Acoustic McCartney" for her. As I

leaned on the counter, I said to her, "Remember that conversation we had last week about McCartney?"

"Oh yeah," she said. "As a matter of fact, my boyfriend and I just got finished rewatching the entire *Beatles Anthology* on video."

"Well," I said, "here's a little mix for you to play while stuck in L.A. traffic or right here at your desk."

"No frickin' way!!!" she said excitedly as she read the song list.

It felt awesome to see her pop awake from her late afternoon slumber in her cubicle and inspect the song list on the CD cover. I had some business to do that I was prepared to pay $20 for, but she wouldn't take my money.

That was completely unexpected. I wasn't looking for any kind of discount, but I guess the simple act of remembering our conversation and following up on it with the CD really made an impression on her. It was a very, very cool interaction for my first gift.

I get up from my computer and do an awkward little happy hop-skip down our hallway, through the dining room and into the closet Mark uses as an office and recording studio. I burst through the door and kiss him. "Thanks, honey!"

He just smiles his cute little grin. He knows why I'm there.

gift 18 ~ Grandma's Gift

I have one grandmother still alive and her eighty-sixth birthday is in seven days. Deciding what present to give her isn't a simple task. Agatha Walker, my father's mother, is a woman who doesn't want for much. She's not wealthy. She lives a humble life and doesn't appreciate extravagances. I always try to give my grandma practical things like wallets or gift certificates for her hairdresser's. She appreciates things she can use, not things that just sit around the house like flowers or knickknacks.

Grandma Walker spent her entire life in central Nebraska. She still manages the family farming operation my grandfather, Floyd Walker, ran until the day he died twelve years ago, though today she rents most of the land to cousins and they plant and harvest the crops. This farmland has been in our family for nearly one hundred years, so a deep respect for hard work and the land is part of my heritage. I grew up spending at least a month every summer with my grandparents and those were some of the happiest times of my life.

My mother's parents, Gladys and William Greathouse, lived just thirty minutes from Grandma and Grandpa Walker, so my two sisters and I rattled back and forth between the two small towns all summer in my Grandma Walker's green Ford Mercury or Grandma Greathouse's blue Buick Century, splitting our time between each side of the family.

My mother's family are not farmers. My grandfather was a carpenter until his hands became crippled by rheumatoid arthritis (yet another autoimmune disease), and my grandmother was primarily a mother. Though they didn't sow crops, both of them were master gardeners. I recall spending hours squatted in the plot behind their house pulling weeds and snitching strawberries and snap peas off the vines. I also used to enjoy sitting in my grandpa's workshop as he fixed things like the transistor radio or the oak footstool that I used to stand on in the kitchen as I helped grandma prepare dinner. I'd wash the garden dirt from the tomatoes that were served fresh, sliced on a plate with every meal. Grandma Greathouse used to play dress up with us, allowing us to pick anything from her closet for our mock beauty pageants and dance contests. My mother's side of the family was small. She had two sisters, but one died at age 18 of cancer. Her other sister, Willa, had two children, so our Greathouse family gatherings were always intimate and tame.

My father's side was another story. He is the oldest of four siblings, two boys and two girls who had three kids each. Walker gatherings were boisterous with twelve grandchildren in the ranks. My cousin Staci is the oldest, but I was always the boss of the crew, even though I was six months younger. Grandma Walker called me "the instigator," because I was the one who came up with the brilliant schemes that got us all in trouble. Once I decided we should form a bucket brigade and transform a large cardboard box into a hot tub in the basement. By the time my grandma came downstairs to investigate, the box was half full of water and had already started to disintegrate. Of course, the basement carpet got soaked. Grandma wasn't thrilled. I remember her trying to scold us, but in the middle of it she started laughing so hard she cried.

Another time, I emptied an entire container of Johnson's baby powder onto the oak floor in my grandma's bedroom. Then I encouraged all of my cousins to join me in an "ice skating" contest in our stocking feet. The powder made the floor a perfect slippery surface and we glided and leaped around for forty-five minutes before my grandma burst into the bedroom to find us all spinning in a huge cloud of white dust. We were covered in powder—and so was the floor and every square inch of furniture in the room.

"I don't want to see any of you outside this door until this mess is cleaned up," she scolded as she slammed the bedroom door shut. This time she wasn't laughing.

It took us three hours to clean up the mess to her satisfaction, but when we had, she took us all out to the Dairy Barn for soft-serve ice cream.

I wonder what I should get her for her birthday this year? I think as I walk to a local shop. *I just got her a wallet for Christmas so that's out.* I wander the aisles until I get to the kitchen section and begin to sort through the dish towels and pot holders. I find a cute set with little roosters and chickens pecking at the ground in a barnyard. It reminds me of spending time with my grandma on the farm.

My two favorite things to do on the farm were to help her prepare meals and go with her to the henhouse to collect eggs. Grandma made three meals a day for my grandfather, all the hired hands, and any number of relatives who happened to be visiting. It wasn't uncommon for her to cook for twenty people and I loved being the sous chef. For lunch, we would tear apart heads of lettuce and shred carrots to make tossed salad in the mint green Tupperware bowl she always used. Or I'd butter bread to help her make stacks and stacks of ham sandwiches. I would peel potatoes, shuck corn, or snap fresh green beans, which she always slow cooked in water with little pieces of bacon.

Each morning, I'd walk along the dirt path to the henhouse, holding my grandma's hand, and we would carefully collect a basket full of eggs from the nests. She would let me crack the eggs into a large bowl to scramble once we were back in the kitchen. While the bacon sizzled and the eggs fried, I would make piles of toast that I would slather with butter and serve with the meal. If I was lucky, I'd get to go out with Grandpa Walker to check irrigation, feed cattle, or ride around on the tractors doing chores. Since there were so many grandkids, we had to take turns going with him. My cousin Staci, my middle sister, Joelle, and I usually went together a few mornings a week. On the way back to the house for lunch, we would always beg my grandpa to stop at the grain elevator so we could all get one of the free lollipops the operators handed out. Then we would insist that he drive us home on what we called "Roller Coaster Road," a hilly dirt road we all loved. Even though it was the long way home, Grandpa always gave in, and we three girls would sit cheering next to him on the bench seat of his red Ford pickup as he sped over the hills with the windows open.

"Wheeeeee! Wheeeeee! Wheeeeee!" we'd yell at the top

of our lungs, our sun-bleached blond hair whipping in the wind. Grandpa would chuckle at us.

A dishtowel and potholder seem like pretty meager offerings for my grandma, of whom I have such fond memories. But I know she'll put these items to good use. When I get home I write out a nice card telling my grandma how much I love and appreciate her. Then I wrap the gift in tissue paper and put it in a box to mail. I smile, imagining her hands opening the gift and thinking of those long-ago summers, too.

gift 19 ~ Celebrating Steps

SUNDAY, APRIL 6

Mark and I pull into the parking lot at the Self-Realization Fellowship Temple fifteen minutes before the meditation service is scheduled to begin. The beauty of the temple is almost overwhelming: the structure is blinding white in the sun and covered in intricate decorative detail, like a mini Taj Mahal. Bright blue stone and tile work is set into the concrete surrounding the manicured grounds, which are beautifully landscaped with a full spectrum of colorful flowers. Because we're on a hill near the coast, we get glimpses of the ocean in a few places as we walk around the temple to the front entrance.

We chat with a woman who is handing out programs. She tells us this land and the construction of the temple were a gift from a devotee of Paramahansa Yogananda, who moved to the U.S. from India and founded the Self-Realization Fellowship. I have read Yogananda's book, *Autobiography of a Yogi,* and have long wanted to attend a service at one of his temples. On entering, we're surprised to see that the interior is rather simple. It's carpeted in blue, and a large oil painting of Yogananda hangs on the altar beside an arrangement of yellow and orange flowers. The room is full of straight-backed wooden chairs, most with occupants already. Mark and I claim two seats in a center row and wait for the service to begin.

The man who leads the service is soft-spoken. We strain to hear him speak and take in his words. He talks of finding peace in the face of chaos. Then we all meditate together. My own meditation is far from peaceful. My "monkey mind" is in full swing, unable to stop racing from thought to thought through the anxiety jungle: *I'm feeling better, but what happens if I crash again? Will I ever be able to have a baby? I should start practicing yoga more regularly again. I can't believe I'm walking almost normally again.*

Each time I notice that I've latched onto a new vine of thinking, I imagine my gold ball of energy in the center of my head and direct all of my attention there. By the end of the twenty-minute meditation, my mind is finally quiet. I feel a small sense of that inner peace the speaker talked of earlier.

Mark and I drop a $5 bill into the collection plate at the end of the service. This is our gift for the day. Then we join the other members of the congregation for "Friendship Tea" after the service and enjoy cups of chai, little samosas, and other pastries. Mark and I sit quietly amid the chatter going on around us, eating and enjoying the aftereffects of our meditation.

After a few minutes, Mark looks at me expectantly. "So, are you feeling up to it?"

"I am. Let's try it."

Mark takes my right arm and we walk through the temple and out a set of French doors to the grounds. A beautiful lake lies behind the temple with more than 100 steps leading down to it.

"Wow. That's a lot of stairs." Mark glances over at me. "Are you sure?"

I feel good, and I haven't thought much about my cane since I lost it last week. "I can do it. I may have to stop and rest a few times, though." I am determined to walk around that lake, but first I have to get down all those stairs.

I descend slowly, gripping the railing on my right side and Mark's arm on my left. I stop three times to steady myself along the way, but make it down the entire set of stairs. I allow myself to feel victorious, pushing aside for now the thought that I'll have to climb back up all of them, a much tougher proposition.

"I did it!" I say to Mark as we step off the final stair and onto the sloped landing that will lead us down to the lake.

Mark beams a triumphant smile back at me. "You did great!"

He takes my hand in his and we begin to walk slowly toward the lake. This is one of the most beautiful places I've ever been. Lily pads and lotus flowers float in the water and every inch of the landscape bursts with greenery and brightly colored flowers. Along the lakeside path, five temples are dedicated to the major religions in the world: Jewish, Hindu, Muslim, Buddhist, Christian. A memorial to Mahatma Gandhi stands as well, where some of his ashes are kept in a crypt. Swans and ducks swim around on the surface of the lake, and we see a family of turtles, several frogs, and schools of orange koi gliding under the surface as we walk. When we reach the end of the path on the other side of the lake, we sit down in a small gazebo so I can rest. We do not speak. We just sit quietly and hold hands for some time. I turn to Mark and thank him. I can't seem to do that enough.

"C'mon babe, you're strong," he says. "And you're determined, not to mention a little stubborn. I mean, once you set your mind to something, nothing stops you. You just don't give up."

I laugh a little at that. Mark is right. My stubbornness tends to serve me well. I inherited this trait from my father, and I believe he got it from my grandma.

"Should we try to tackle the stairs again?" asks Mark as he stands and reaches down to help me up.

"I don't need help. I can do it," I say, pushing myself off the bench.

"See what I mean? You're damn stubborn." A laugh is threaded through his words.

"Let's go," I say, and start off toward the stairs on my own.

When we get to the base of the stairs, I gape, bug-eyed, at the tower of steps before me.

"How do you want to do this?" asks Mark.

"By myself," I tell him, "but with you behind me so you can catch me if I fall." We proceed in this way, stopping five times along the way so I can rest. It's a long, slow haul, and by the time we make it to the top my legs are shaky and my lungs burn.

"Right on! You did it!" Mark says, sitting beside me on a bench.

"Good thing I'm stubborn," I say, then I lean into him and begin to cry quietly. He puts his arm around me and lets me weep out my relief.

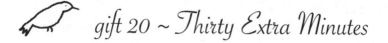

gift 20 ~ Thirty Extra Minutes

I'm tired today. I anticipated this reaction to yesterday's mountain of stairs, so I didn't schedule anything for myself until late afternoon. When I feel an urge to push myself to get up and get going with my day, I recall Mbali's early warning: "Don't push yourself to the point that you feel depleted."

I stay in bed, alternating between sleeping and reading until I take a prearranged call in the afternoon from a new client. Simla, a personal nutrition coach, has booked me for one hour. We are on a roll with marketing ideas after forty-five minutes, so I offer to extend the call to ninety minutes at no additional charge. This little gift is offered out of my gratitude to be working again.

Simla happily accepts the free thirty minutes and goes on to tell me about some of her business name ideas. My favorite from her possibilities is *Delicious Health*. The vibrant name matches the level of enthusiasm Simla brings to her work. But she is really stuck when it comes to her tagline, despite the two pages of ideas she e-mailed me before our call. Simla specializes in working with people who are living overstressed lives and beginning to suffer health challenges because of it—something I can certainly identify with. In the decade-plus that I spent working in advertising before my

MS diagnosis, the hours were long, the work was intense, and I lived from deadline to deadline.

I remember once working three days straight with no sleep on a big pitch for a large international account. On the third day, I fainted in the design studio. One of the art directors came running through the maze of cubes when she heard me hit the floor. She grabbed a stack of layout sheets and began frantically waving them back and forth over my face to give me some air. Somehow I managed to pick myself up off the floor and write the last few headlines we needed to finish the presentation in time for our five o'clock deadline. Then I went into my office, crawled underneath my desk and slept for three hours. I was too tired to even go home.

People who are attracted to the deadline-driven world of advertising are adrenaline junkies. I got a sick thrill out of pushing myself past my limits almost every day. Looking back now, I can see that each time I did so I was overriding my nervous system, which couldn't have helped my condition. Even back then, I was experiencing numerous symptoms that I now know are MS-related. Add to the mix the sugar, carb, and caffeine-fueled diet I existed on during those years and you have a recipe for the disaster I became. Knowing now that stress is a major factor in autoimmune diseases, I understand that I might not have crossed the line into full-blown MS if I had made different lifestyle choices.

Simla wants to teach people how to use food as medicine and make lifestyle changes so they can live healthy, balanced lives. She came to her new career in nutrition after burning herself out as a management consultant—traveling constantly, rubbing elbows with bigwigs, making lots of money, and working in very high pressure situations. There are many parallels between our stories, though in her case, a different autoimmune disease—fibromyalgia—brought her to her knees. Just like me, Simla's body broke down and demanded she limp away from her high-powered career and rebirth her life. After much exploration, she learned to manage her condition through nutrition and lifestyle, and now she wants to help other people avoid pushing themselves into the types of health conditions she and I live with.

"How about, *Healthy eating for busy bodies?*" I suggest. "Or *Healthy eating for balanced being?*" These are slight variations on taglines she already has on her long list of ideas.

"Those aren't bad," she replies. I can tell by her tone she's not thrilled.

"Don't worry," I reassure her, leaning forward in my chair as if she's right in front of me. "We'll come up with something that feels right. But I have a question. Do you think you're really feeling stuck over your tagline, or is there something deeper going on?"

Like all my clients, Simla originally called me for help on her branding, website, and other marketing materials—but I've learned after watching nearly fifty women start businesses that a successful launch has little to do with what shade of green you decide on for your logo or what five words you choose for your tagline. The things that limit most of us from moving forward are emotional blocks that boil down to fear, uncertainty, and doubt.

"You're right," Simla admits tentatively. "It's not really about the tagline. I'm scared I'll spend a lot of money, energy, and time to get my business off the ground and fall into the same tendency to overwork that led me to this place to begin with. I don't want to work myself sick again."

Now we're getting to the root of why, with all the strong candidates on her list, Simla is resisting making a tagline decision. I suggest that we switch gears for a while. Sometimes I like to use guided meditation with clients. I talk her through some techniques intended to help her ground herself and release fear. Then I teach her a few simple meditations that often bring people a greater sense of clarity. I've spent a long time learning and teaching these complex exercises, but I put them into simple enough terms for her to follow my instructions.

"Oh my God, I feel so much better," says Simla at the end of the twenty-minute visualization.

Before we hang up, Simla books several more sessions and I give her a list of action steps I'd like her to complete before we talk again. One of them is to go out into nature and look for inspiration for logo symbols. Another is to practice some of the visualizations I taught her for at least five minutes every day. I feel certain that she'll follow through and that by our next call, Simla will have settled on a tagline and be ready to begin giving her new company a voice that will resonate strongly in the world.

I unplug my headset and say a quick prayer of gratitude. Then I spin around in my office chair, thrilled to be back in business and connecting with my clients again. Working with women who are in the seedling stage of businesses is so much more meaningful and fulfilling to me than writing junk mail packages and spam for the corporate giants who were my clients during my ad agency days.

I wonder if the recent windfall of business I've experienced is a result of my giving, I find myself thinking, and immediately feel ashamed of the thought. It almost feels unfair that I've received so much more than I've given. *Do I really deserve all this good fortune?* I recognize my old foes—guilt and self-deprecation—jumping to the forefront of my mind, and immediately reframe the thought.

"I deserve good fortune," I say out loud to my office walls.

I've come to believe over the last twenty days that giving and receiving are two sides of the same coin. One cannot exist without the other. I now view giving and receiving as an exchange of energy—a universal transaction that each one of us takes part in over and over, moment to moment. I am also seeing that each exchange—whether I am on the giving or the receiving end—is a divine experience, what my mother would call a God Moment. During the moments I am offering or accepting a gift, the part of me that is true spirit is connecting with the true spirit of another individual, and we are both in that instant connected to the divine force that created everything out of nothing, the light from which we all draw inspiration and energy.

I have been meditating regularly since Day 6 of my giving experiment. I don't always remember to begin my day with a specific affirmation, as Mbali suggested, but I have been praying each day in addition to my meditation practice. The prayer I say each morning is one I devised years ago:

Namo Guru Dev Namo. (*Sanskrit for "I call upon the e."*) I offer my efforts before you, the teacher who is formless and supreme. May I be a channel of your will and your love. Guide me today in service of you and my fellows.

This revival of my spiritual practice has resulted in what my mentors and teachers over the years have called God Consciousness—a deeper personal relationship with spirit. For me, the daily prayer and meditation have restored a sense of purpose, something I was missing during the dark free-falling months of illness that preceded my first day of giving. What I can clearly see now is that I turned the lights off myself and leapt out of the plane without my parachute. God was there the whole time, ready to catch me. All I had to do was acknowledge the presence of this universal spirit and open my eyes to the light.

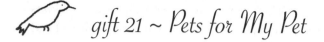 *gift 21 ~ Pets for My Pet*

TUESDAY, APRIL 8

Eve's new design for the Giving Challenge website is beautiful, featuring a tree sprouting leaves with birds nesting in it. She tells me that the tree is symbolic of rebirth and revitalization and the birds symbolize freedom and liberation of spirit. I didn't provide her with any creative direction and I'm amazed that she has come up with something so perfectly aligned with Mbali's nature-based philosophies. It's exciting to know we'll have the freshly designed website live sometime in the next week, likely around the time I give my twenty-ninth gift.

I log on to read some of the stories written by the now fifty-seven people who have joined the site and begun posting their gift-giving tales. Most are people I'm happy to be reconnecting with: old friends from Nebraska, where I grew up and went to college, plus friends, clients, and mentors from my decade in the San Francisco Bay Area. Some of my family members are also taking part now. My mom is giving daily and blogging about her experiences. My sister Joelle, Ryan (my unofficial brother-in-law), and their two children are all giving. A couple of cousins have signed up and started giving. A few friends of friends have begun signing up now, too. It's fun to see names of people I don't know personally.

Most of the stories people post on the site are simple

accounts of what they've given. One woman tells of writing her mother a letter and mailing it to her with a book. A man tells of helping a friend clean out her garage. Another woman took a friend from work out to lunch. Three different people write that giving feels easy to them; the challenge lies in offering the gifts consciously rather than just in passing. I agree that it's sometimes hard to stop for a few seconds *before* offering the gift to consider where it is coming from. Am I offering it out of gratitude, joy, and a true desire to share something with another person? Or is there a sense of obligation lurking under the surface or a desire to get something back? Many of us yearn to experience moments of true altruism—where we're authentically offering a gift out of a simple, honest desire to do something nice for someone and expecting nothing in return.

People also seem to be struggling a bit with what "counts" as a gift.

"I read a bedtime story to my son last night, but that doesn't count because I do that every night anyway," writes one woman.

"Smiles are easy for me to give, as are words of advice. I want to use this 29 Days to go deeper and offer things I wouldn't normally give," writes another.

One of the profound changes I've seen for myself since I began giving is that I now feel comfortable counting every gift I mindfully offer to another person. I no longer feel pressure to make a grand gesture for it to count.

The words of advice I offer a client. The dishes I decide to wash instead of leaving them for Mark. The spare change I decide to drop in the tip jar at the coffee shop or hand to the stranger on the street. These are all gifts. For me, this is a fundamental shift in mindset that has resulted in a greater sense of freedom and joy. If I wash the dishes because "I'm supposed to" or make suggestions to a client because "I have to," I am in a very different mind space when taking the action. I actually end up feeling resentful. When I'm approaching everything as a gift, my heart feels open and it's easier to enjoy my day, my life. Smiles are much easier to come by. Giggles burst forth unexpectedly. Sometimes I find myself dancing to imaginary music in my head. I can't imagine anyone ever telling a person diagnosed with MS to "lighten up," but that's exactly what I've done and I feel so much better for it.

Others who are sharing on the website have issues with receiving.

"I think I need a do-over," writes one woman. "I actually received from others in Days 8 and 9, which was a little weird for me. Maybe my giving challenge turned into a receiving challenge (which is a challenge for certain). I am going to give three things today, which is Day 9."

I can now see that part of Mbali's intention with this prescription was to help me learn the art of receiving. Many of us are programmed to resist life's gifts. Even the Bible tells us in Acts 20:35, "It's better to give than to receive."

There is certainly an exchange of power involved in giving and receiving. For some reason, the receiver is often seen as "lesser than." I suppose because they're the one in need of assistance. It's widely accepted that giving is empowering, but I've learned in the past three weeks that opening myself up to receive freely is just as energizing and fulfilling.

My back is starting to hurt pretty bad, so I turn my computer off. I feel a deep sense of fulfillment knowing that this little experiment seems to be having a positive impact on many of the people I love most in the world. We are learning things about ourselves through this exercise. Mbali would say, "We are making conscious connections with other people, which makes life *feel* more purposeful, therefore it is."

I lie down on the couch in my office and prop my head on a pillow. Habib, my little cat who has been keeping me company, flops herself down on the floor nearby. Most of her body is covered in striped gray patterns, but the area around her nose, chin, belly, and all four paws is pure white. She has huge gold eyes and always looks like she's got a little smile on her face, which earned her the nickname "Disney Kitty" from one of my old roommates. I reach down and give Habib a good scratch behind her little gray ears. "How are you, Disney Kitty?" I coo as I pet the top of her silky head. She flips herself over, belly up, and I smile as she wiggles her little kitty body around on the rug, leaving clumps of gray hair in her wake.

My gift for the day will be a good belly rub for Habib. I reach down and begin to rub under her chin and work my way down to the middle of her white furry belly, where she loves to be petted the most. She closes her eyes and throws her head back in ecstasy, purring loudly to encourage me to keep going. When the belly rub is complete, she climbs up on the couch, curls up next to me, and we both doze off, companions in a cat nap.

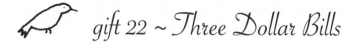

gift 22 ~ Three Dollar Bills

It is 7:30 p.m. and I am arriving at a women's addiction support meeting, feeling distracted and drained. I had phone sessions with two clients today—the first time I have worked with two people in one day—and I think it was too much. As soon as I sit down on the cold metal folding chair that will be my nest for the next hour, it occurs to me that I have not given a gift today.

I mentally review my day to see if there's anything I can count as a gift after the fact. I made a smoothie for breakfast and shared it with Mark. I called my mom earlier today just to say hello and check in. I let one of the client sessions run an extra fifteen minutes without charge. *I just decided yesterday that everything counts, right?* But one of the points of this exercise is to practice mindfulness . . . to offer each gift with a sense of consciousness and intention. It's true that I did a number of nice things for others today, but I didn't do them with the conscious intention of giving.

Oh shit, I'm going to have to start over at Day 1 tomorrow. I recall this instruction from Mbali from the day she gave me this prescription—to begin again at the beginning if I forget one day. I feel a deep sense of disappointment and dread about the idea of starting again—like I failed a test and now have to take it again. The perfectionist in me is not happy at all about this possibility.

The day isn't over, I tell myself. *Maybe there's someone here I can give to.*

I look around at all the well-put-together women in this circle and am at a loss. Most of them have been sober for a year or more, while I am back in my first thirty days of sobriety—I started over after detoxing off the recent round of drugs. One of the primary principles of recovery from addiction is honesty, so I had to admit that I'd been taking more of a number of the medications than I was prescribed. It was humbling to show up at these meetings and admit that I was no longer "five years sober." Here I sit, looking slightly unkempt in a pair of old sweat pants and my favorite Supergirl T-shirt. I haven't even showered today—I just didn't have the energy. The women in this room speak of having jobs and children and lives that have been rebuilt in sobriety with hard work and commitment, one day at a time. They all seem to represent the woman I want to be when I grow up, and I don't feel there's anything I could offer a single one of them at this moment.

Maybe I can give one of them a compliment, I think, getting preoccupied with my mission instead of paying attention to the meeting. *No, that would be contrived.*

I grab my purse and shuffle through its contents, disrupting the people near me. There is nothing in here to pass on. None of these women want my $8 gas-station sunglasses or a six-month-old tin of Altoids.

Then the leader of the meeting saves me.

She passes around a basket to collect cash to help cover

the meeting's expenses. I often ignore this basket and shamefully pass it on to the next person without adding any money to the collection. This time, I dig my wallet out of my bag and pull out all the cash I have—three $1 bills. I drop them in the hot pink plastic basket when the woman next to me hands it over. Disappointed, I begin to paw through my purse again, wishing for $5 or $10. Three dollars just doesn't seem like enough—which is a direct reflection of how I'm feeling about myself in this moment: *I'm not enough.*

I have spent the last thirty minutes in a completely self-centered conversation with myself, which has left me feeling alone while sitting in a room full of other people. I have forgotten that I am a part of this circle of women, and that we're all here for a common purpose: to help one another stay sober. I take another look around the room and realize that nobody here is judging me . . . in fact, many of the women make eye contact with me and smile as I scan their faces.

While I was busy comparing our outsides, I lost sight of what we have in common on the inside. Most drug addicts and alcoholics share a chronic sense of self-loathing—what many of us see as a gaping hole in our spirits that we attempt to fill with booze or pills or powders. There is a deep sense of lack in an addict's world—there's never enough of anything we think we need to be happy, including self-esteem, love, and attention. When we get sober we begin to practice self-love, many of us for the first time. For most of us, loving ourselves is like asking a fish to grow legs—it just doesn't feel natural.

I genuinely want to support this meeting. It has been a respite for me in the last few weeks. *Those three dollars will help buy a box of hot chocolate for the next meeting,* I tell myself. *I just helped ensure the meeting stays operational for others like me who need help staying sober. My intention is what makes my gift matter, not the dollar amount.*

I try to remember that perfection is not expected of me with this giving ritual—or with any other part of my life. *I am enough, just as I am.* I am reminded that the gifts we choose to offer make a difference in the world and connect us to the divine spirit that unites us all. Yes, Mbali did suggest starting over if I forget a day, but she didn't mean it as a form of punishment to punctuate failure.

"The important thing is not to quit," I recall her saying. "Energy will build over the 29 Days. If you forget a day, you will release the energy by starting over and then it will begin to rebuild when you start with Day 1 again. If starting over is too much for you to handle, just begin the next day where you left off."

I certainly feel the energy building for me. The three-dollar contribution has left me feeling chipper enough to talk to a few of the women after the meeting. One of them, Christal, invites me out to dinner with a small group who get together after each week's meeting. A month ago I would have wanted to slink away after the meeting and go home to sleep. Now, I'm feeling pleased that I've helped defray the costs of these meetings, and I'm chatting with Christal as though I've known her for years.

gift 23 ~ Special Shell

I settle into my meditation chair, bare feet planted firmly on the chilly wood floor. I often like to hold something while I meditate, so today I reach out and take one of the shells off the small table next to my chair, a small, coral-colored conch shell about two inches long. It is perfectly intact, spiraling outward into a small point on each end without a single crack. I found this shell while walking on a beach in Florida eight years ago.

I envision myself sitting in a bubble of gold energy, which for me represents my highest spiritual state. I feel a sense of peace and serenity settle in as I reflect on gratitude. An image of Dr. Kim's smiling face pops into my mind.

After my meditation, I prepare some gifts for her. She has helped me so much the past couple of months. Thanks to her daily massages, acupuncture treatments, and icky-tasting herbal "teas"—not to mention her generous rides to and from my appointments—I am now having regular bowel movements and my pain is manageable. At my first appointment, it hurt every time I moved. The pain in my back was a constant searing burn that would leave me writhing in bed crying my eyes out. My feet often hurt so bad it was sometimes impossible for me to put any weight on them to walk. I also used to have horrible constipation, which made me feel nauseated and bloated.

I open the kitchen cupboard where I keep a vast array of herbal teas and pull out a few bags of each flavor. I find an empty glass canister and arrange the teabags inside in a colorful pattern. I'm also going to give Dr. Kim my little conch shell because I know she will appreciate it.

In Hindu tradition, conch shells are used for ritualistic purposes. The conch is blown as a ceremonial horn during worship. The God of Preservation, Vishnu, is often depicted holding a conch that represents life. In the Buddhist tradition—which Dr. Kim practices—the conch shell is considered one of the Eight Auspicious Symbols. The resonating sound of the conch shell being blown represents the universal, penetrating spiritual calling of the Buddha, which can awaken us from ignorance and urges us to succeed with our own welfare and assist in the welfare of others. It seems to me that Dr. Kim has answered this calling and is a wonderful example of this principle in living action.

I put the tea and the shell into a small paper shopping bag with some cheerful lavender and green tissue paper.

Dr. Kim looks thrilled when I hand her the bag. The room hums with an orderly, Zen energy. Three beautiful flower arrangements rest on the shelves behind her desk, one with orange and yellow roses and two with different types of orchids. Judging from the little cards sticking out of the pots, these are all office-warming gifts from patients.

Dr. Kim dips her hands into the bag and pulls out the first item, her sweet smile beaming. She takes time to examine each flavor of tea, curious about the ingredients in the blends. She rolls her office chair over to a small table next to her desk and pushes a button on her electric teapot to heat up some water.

"We have tea after treatment," she says as she plucks two bags of licorice-mint tea out of the canister.

Next, she unwraps the little shell.

"Oh. Is very special! Many thanks," she says as she turns the shell over and over, examining it from all angles. She reaches into the shelves behind her desk and picks up a small wooden box with a black and white yin yang symbol on top of it. She opens the box and I see that the inside is lined with soft, royal-blue fabric. She gently places the shell inside and closes the lid. *What a graceful recipient,* I think. *She's clearly already learned the reciprocal connection between giving and receiving.*

Reciprocity is an important principle in most Asian cultures. It is common practice in Korean culture to reciprocate gifts with more gifts, and giving gifts is part of the basic philosophy of how people are expected to treat one another. In Western Christian culture the practice of reciprocity is commonly called The Golden Rule. One of the first bible verses I remember learning in Sunday School is, "Do unto others as you would have them do unto you" (Luke 6:31).

Sociologists and psychologists often use the concept of reciprocity to explain altruism. They say our expectation is that helping others will increase the possibility that they will help us in the future. The human desire to reciprocate kindness is one of the things that I have come to believe enables us to coexist. I think, for most of us, the practice of reciprocity is intrinsic to our social conditioning. It is a "natural" behavior and one of the things that earns us the label of human beings.

Dr. Kim and I exchange many thank-yous back and forth. We both have goofy smiles on our faces as we step into the treatment room and I climb onto her table. I lie face down. As usual, she starts by rubbing my feet in fast, deep strokes. She digs her fingers into the arches of my feet and my heels, making me squirm. Then she begins to knead into my calves, which hurts a lot. These daily Tui Na massages are not the type of relaxing, put-you-to-sleep massages you would get at a spa. They hurt. With each deep stroke, I let out a little yelp of pain. Dr. Kim calls out the organ associated with the area she's kneading. Ovaries. Kidneys. Liver. Spleen. Intestines. Apparently most of my organs are not in perfect harmony or the massages wouldn't hurt so much.

After the massage, Dr. Kim inserts her needles. Most acupuncture needles are very fine—some as fine as a human hair—so most people feel no pain when they are inserted. Because I've been in her care for a few months now, Dr. Kim has begun to use bigger, more powerful needles that she inserts more deeply. I feel a little zing of pain as each needle goes in, which quickly subsides and gives way to an almost hypnotic sense of calm. Next, Dr. Kim lights a stick of moxa—which looks kind of like a black cigar—and waves the warm herby-scented stick over various parts of my body. This soothes me, and I fall asleep on the table. She wakes me up to remove the needles and then brings me a cup of the tea she has prepared. I deeply inhale its minty scent as I take my first sip.

When I exit the treatment room and go back into her office, Dr. Kim jumps up from her desk and scampers over to a table near the door. She picks up a flat, arrow-shaped brown stone that is quite large—maybe five inches across—and has points and knobs sticking out from its edges. She reaches out and hands it to me. The stone has some weight to it and is perfectly polished.

"Cami. This is special massage stone I am giving to you," says Dr. Kim. She guides my hand holding the stone and shows me the various places I should massage on my head, neck, and shoulders every day.

I feel a bubble of discomfort form in my belly . . . and for a moment I consider saying, *Oh no, you don't need to give me this just because I brought you something today.*

But I know this is not the response that will make Dr. Kim feel good. Instead, I say, "Thank you. I'll use it every day and think of you."

gift 24 ~ Planting Thanks

I'm happy to see a bunch of names I don't recognize on the 29 Gifts website when I log on. There are now 103 committed givers, nearly twice the number who were signed up just a few days ago! The new ones have been led here by a woman named Britt Bravo, who has sent me an e-mail explaining that she wrote about the 29-Day Giving Challenge on her own blog. Britt's story triggers a number of other bloggers to write about the Challenge on their sites throughout the day, and another thirty-one people sign up before I leave my house in the afternoon for my walk. This ritual has made such a huge impact on my life, and I'm happy to be able to share it with others.

Today I have an appointment for a massage at Grace Healing Center near my house, so instead of walking my laps around the block, I walk to a grocery store nearby to purchase some flowers for Grace Ko, the center's owner, as my gift for the day. Grace has been giving me massages once a week for a few months now, which has really helped reduce the amount of pain I live with.

I wander around the small flower department until I find a display of plants covered in little hot pink blooms. I recall that Grace has lots of plants growing in her waiting area, so she must have a greener thumb than I do. Now she'll have a new one to tend.

A few people on the 29 Gifts website have been writing about their "stealth gives." One woman put a gift basket in the women's restroom where she works. Another, who is a writer, has been leaving copies of her book on park benches and buses with notes on them that say, "For you to enjoy." Some people believe that giving anonymously is more honorable and spiritually rewarding. Some of them quote Matthew 6:2–4 as evidence that gifts should be offered anonymously: *So when you give to the needy, do not announce it with trumpets . . . to be honored by men. I tell you the truth, they have received their reward in full. But when you give to the needy, do not let your left hand know what your right hand is doing, so that your giving may be in secret. Then your Father, who sees what is done in secret, will reward you.*

"It has been my experience that secret giving is much more powerful, and to give and not be found out is harder because you must be humble to not get pats on the back for what you are doing," wrote one woman on the site.

Personally, I don't believe that a gift must be kept secret for it to be transformational and powerful. At least not for the purpose of this particular giving ritual, which is more about mindfulness and developing a conscious habit of reaching out to others. For me, writing about my gifts each day has kept giving top of mind. I also appreciate the others who are writing about their giving experiences because it inspires me to keep giving. But I do think it would be fun to try to plant my thanks at Grace's Healing Center today without being found out.

When I arrive, all the practitioners are working on clients, which gives me the perfect opportunity to leave my gift unnoticed on the coffee table in the lounge area. There are so many plants in this room, they may not even notice the new addition.

A few minutes later, Grace comes into the lounge and immediately begins to coo over the little plant. She comments that the bright pink blooms match one of the stripes in the shirt I am wearing. With my weak poker face, she figures out immediately that I am the flower fairy. No stealth gives today, but I smile and accept her words of thanks.

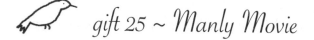 *gift 25 ~ Manly Movie*

SATURDAY, APRIL 12

Mark and I are giving each other the gift of spending time together today. He's been so busy that it feels like we don't
connect for days at a time—great for his business, but not so
great for our marriage. He's really hustling to get his voice-
acting career rolling in L.A., which requires a lot of driving
all over the sprawling metropolis to hit auditions, network-
ing events, and recording gigs. It'll get even more intense
soon when he starts auditioning for on-camera television
commercials in addition to all his voiceover work.

We debate for a while what to do on our date day. We
agree we want to see a movie but can't agree on which one.
I'm pretty pushy, and we typically have a verbal wrestling
match over the TV remote, let alone a movie. I almost always
win, just because I'm more stubborn than Mark. Here's my
chance for today's gift.

"You choose," I offer.

He gives me a suspicious look. "What?"

"Seriously," I reassure him. "It's your pick. I promise I'll
go to any movie you pick and I won't complain."

Taking full advantage, he suggests *Leatherheads,* a period
film starring George Clooney and Renée Zellweger that doc-
uments the beginning of professional American football.

Mark knows that I hate period films—and that I hate sports even more.

"OK. *Leatherheads*," I concur, but he knows the cheer I'm forcing into my voice is fake. *At least George Clooney is hot,* I say to myself. *And I liked Renée Zellweger a lot in* Bridget Jones's Diary *and* Jerry Maguire.

I haven't taken my walk today yet, so we set out on foot to Grauman's Chinese Theater, not far from our house. Though I've often passed by it, this is my first time inside this Hollywood landmark, where all the big movie premieres are held. It's beautiful inside. I especially love the ladies' lounge, which has all of the original art deco decor, including the ornate mirrors. Those mirrors have seen some very famous faces. *Maybe Bette Davis or Ingrid Bergman looked in this mirror,* I think as I lean in to apply a fresh coat of lip gloss.

The film isn't bad. There's some comedy and girlie romance thrown in along with the manly grunting and butting heads on the football field, which makes it tolerable.

When we get home, I make us a simple dinner to give Mark a break from kitchen duty. I throw some chicken breasts into a marinade of soy sauce, rice vinegar, and ginger, put some rice in the rice cooker, and steam some broccoli, Mark's favorite vegetable.

After we enjoy our meal, I surprise Mark with the biggest gift of the day.

"You can have control of the remote tonight," I say. "We'll watch anything you want."

Mark is in heaven as he selects *The Daily Show* from our Tivo and kicks back to watch it without a peep of protest from me. I'm only half-watching, thinking how good it feels to release control of things, even little things like this. I get to see Mark happy. It feels good not to fight about things that don't matter much. Digging in my heels just keeps me rooted to the spot. That's not a position I want to be in.

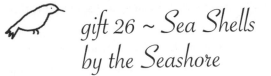

gift 26 ~ Sea Shells by the Seashore

SUNDAY, APRIL 13

I come back from my morning walk to a nice surprise: Mark has cooked us a lovely brunch. I see a platter of pancakes and a bowl of steaming scrambled eggs in the center of the dining room table and two places set for us when I arrive home, sweating from the exertion and the L.A. heat, which is blistering today. He has even folded the cloth napkins into cute little fan shapes. There's warm maple syrup and peanut butter on the table—Mark knows I can't eat pancakes unless they are slathered with both. I compliment all the care he has taken in putting the meal together, and we sit down to enjoy it.

"I'm so impressed. These pancakes are really fluffy," I say after my first bite of sweet, nutty flapjack.

"I whipped the egg whites with the hand blender before adding them to the batter," replies Mark. "I saw the tip on someone's blog."

"These are the best pancakes you've ever made."

We devour the food and then sit chatting for a while as Mark drinks his coffee and I sip my chamomile tea. After our meal, Mark tosses a blanket, some sunscreen, and our books into a duffel bag for a trip to Santa Monica Beach. He also makes us sandwiches and packs them into a little red cooler along with some granola bars, two apples, and several bottles of water.

After the drive, we're pleased that the weather is agreeable by the water. It is nearly 90 degrees and the sun is a blazing burst of light in the cloudless blue sky. Even though spring just started, it already feels like summer. After over a decade living in San Francisco, we're programmed to dress in layers of clothing and be prepared for rain at any moment. But in Los Angeles, the sun comes out every day. It's definitely one of the positive aspects of making the move south.

We slather our pasty white bodies with sunscreen and then spend nearly two hours reclined in the sand on our orange and blue cotton blanket. It's so hot that we brave the frosty water for a while together, but the waves are too much for me. Each time the water ebbs toward the shore or flows back out to sea, I lose my footing and take a tumble into the gently rocking surf. Mark patiently helps me up each time, but I give up and head back to the blanket after three falls. I'd rather be hot than get swept out to sea.

Mark stays in the water for quite some time, splashing around just like the 8-year-old kids who are in the water with him. I laugh as he follows the lead of two little blond surfer boys by attempting to body surf on his middle-aged, slightly paunchy belly. He tries his best to ride the waves, launching his entire body into the surf headfirst again and again. Each time he travels just a few feet before the wave tumbles over his body and leaves him bobbing behind. I can't help but laugh out loud.

After Mark tires from his water sports and dries himself off, we sit and nibble our lunch, read a little, then take a walk along the shore. I pick up a handful of pretty, pebble-size shells that reflect shades of pink and lavender in the sunlight. The air smells salty and a cool breeze has begun to blow in off the water. I pocket my little treasures, planning on putting them on my altar at home. When we return to our blanket to pack up, I notice a cute little girl, about 4 years old, building a sand castle. Her curly blond hair flying in the wind, she focuses intently on filling a pail with wet sand for a new tower.

I exchange a few pleasantries with her mom, who is helping the little girl dig.

"Your daughter is adorable. What's her name?"

"This is Rachel," says the mom. She gives Rachel's back a little pat with one of her sandy hands. I wait until the little girl finishes packing the sand hard into her little lime-green pail and looks up at me.

"Do you like sea shells?" I ask.

"Yes!" She jumps up and steps over the moat she has clearly spent a good amount of time digging.

"Would you like some to decorate your castle with?"

"Sure!" Out pops her open right hand.

There are too many shells to fit in her tiny palm, so she makes a cup with both hands and I fill them with my bounty.

"Thanks." She smiles and turns back to her work . . . I watch as her mother helps her use the shells to outline the shape of a large, arching door on the front of the castle. They carefully set them into place, one at a time.

As Mark and I walk back to the car, we both comment on how amazingly cute Rachel was.

"It was awesome to see her so completely tickled and thrilled to receive some simple sea shells," Mark says as he helps me into the car.

"I know," I reply. "I felt 4 years old again seeing her smile."

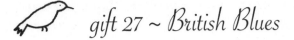
gift 27 ~ British Blues

Eve's new design goes live today and I am thrilled with what she's done. The site feels fresh and light—exactly what I was hoping for. As I type up an e-mail message to blast to all 144 givers, I begin to feel anxious. I'm not sure why, so I step back to think.

For me, anxiety always stems from fear, so I ask myself what I'm afraid of. A number of thoughts come up in answer to the query. *What happens if this thing takes off? I can only work two hours a day. There's no way I'll be able to manage a large online community by myself.*

I realize that months of not working has made me afraid of success on a big scale. The MS flare I'm currently recovering from was largely a result of stress from trying to keep up with the quick growth of my consulting business. I am worried that I don't know my own limits and I don't want to push myself too hard. *The escalation of the flare was also a result of our decision to move to Los Angeles so quickly,* I remind myself. *I uprooted myself from my support system in San Francisco without making sure I had the proper support in place in our new city.* Once again, I'm stuck in scarcity thinking—"not enough."

I now have a good support system here in Los Angeles. My neurologist, psychiatrist, and acupuncturist are all in my corner. I have a fantastic yoga teacher. Grace does amazing massage and body work. A wonderful chiropractor just joined my team as well. Even more important, I've begun to make some real friends—Christal, Ingrid, and a few other women from my addiction support meetings. I no longer feel completely reliant on Mark for support, which has freed up a lot of energy in our relationship. He's not my caretaker, but my partner again. We've made love three times this month, after having no sex for the previous six months. I didn't have the energy to even think about it.

I talk myself through my fear. If the project grows, the right people will show up to support me. I already have Mbali's pledge of support, and Mark is always willing to help me with things on the computer. Eve and Jeff would be willing to help, too.

Then a new fear arises. *I'm not sure I can tell the world personal details about my health struggles.* I know I will need to openly share my story—all of it, not just the good parts—in order for people to identify and believe this exercise might help them in their own lives. After taking down my old blog, I vowed that I would not go back to living my personal life in public because it invites criticism. Revealing myself in this way again makes me nervous, but I feel strongly that the sacrifice I will make to my own privacy will be worth the good that can come from this project.

I also have an underlying fear about not knowing how everything will unfold. I am a planner. In my work helping people strategize business and marketing plans, I always stress the importance of having a written plan. Back in my ad agency days, we considered the planning stage of a campaign the most crucial part of any project. I don't even go to the grocery store without a detailed shopping list.

But I don't have a plan for this project—I'm just doing the next thing that feels right and seeing what happens. Having some kind of plan would make me feel better. Yet this project is different from any past venture I have involved myself with. I'm not approaching it as a business. It's a creative experiment, and the unplanned nature is part of its appeal. I just want to put something out there and watch what unfolds from it.

I know that fear is the number-one thing that holds us back from taking risks in life and pursuing our dreams. I coach my clients through their fear all the time. I know that if I allow myself to be consumed by these fears, this project will die before it has a chance to live.

After a moment I realize I'm getting ahead of myself. Right now, I'm just writing an e-mail. I'm nervous because I don't know many of these people personally, but it's not a big deal. Just as I teach my clients to do, I visualize all of my fear swirling out of my head, down my spine, and out of my body like I'm flushing a toilet. Then I send the e-mail message without even rereading it, just to get past my fear of moving forward:

Hi There Fellow 29Givers,

First I want to say "WELCOME" to the new people who joined the 29-Day Giving Challenge recently.

We now have 144 Committed Givers and I couldn't be more excited.

I am on Day 27 of my personal challenge and just can't believe all of the things that have happened so far.

When I started my challenge, I wanted to see what would happen in my life if I focused my energy on giving for 29 days. What space would it create for new and unexpected things to occur? What shifts would I see in my thinking and behavior as a result? These were just two of the many questions I was curious about in the beginning, but there's no way I could have anticipated what has unfolded for me.

By Day 27, I am astounded by the magical and miraculous shifts in my life:

* I am feeling happier, healthier, and more in awe with life.
* I find myself smiling and laughing more and more every day.
* My body is stronger and I am recovering from the MS flare that has plagued me for months—I was even able to stop walking with my cane by the end of week two.
* My business has exploded with new opportunities.
*I have started reconnecting with my amazing community of friends and family, people I had been pushing away out of fear since my MS diagnosis.
*I am beginning to form a community of new friends and clients in Los Angeles after feeling isolated here in my new home for several months.
*I am experiencing deeper intimacy in my relationship with my husband.

And this is only the beginning.

As you share your stories online this week, let us know what's coming to you as well as what you're giving.

Peace and light to you all!

Good giving today,

Cami Walker

Now it's time for today's gift. I've been meaning to send this gift all month, but kept putting it off because this one requires a collaborative effort between me and Mark. I asked him to make me a cool mix of songs from British artists to send to my friend Ingrid. I hope that receiving this mixed CD in the mail unexpectedly will give her something to smile about and fondly remind her of home. It includes *This Is England* by The Clash, *One Step Beyond* by Madness, and the *Benny Hill* theme song.

I select one of my mother's wonderful handmade cards and write Ingrid a nice note to accompany the CD. The card I pick has a gold crown on the front, which reminds me of the Queen of England, and it has the word "FRIENDS" boldly printed across a polka-dot background. I mentally send a little prayer to Ingrid: *God, please help Ingrid make peace with her mother's death. Please help her move forward with her own life in honor of her mom.* I can almost see Ingrid dancing in her living room to the mix of songs Mark put together just for her.

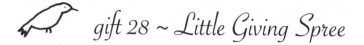 *gift 28 ~ Little Giving Spree*

After twenty-seven days of giving I look forward to watching each day unfold, instead of feeling like a prisoner in my own home. One thing I've noticed with my gifts so far is how it deepens the sense of intimacy I feel with people . . . even people I don't know, like the homeless, drunken stranger I gave 72 cents to. My interactions with the people I choose to give to are so much more meaningful than the day-to-day niceties I've experienced with people in the past. When I am approaching someone with the intention of sharing a small piece of myself—a gift from my heart to theirs—it shifts the dynamic of our communication because I'm showing up to be of service to someone else. I let go of any expectation I may have of them and am just present with them in that moment.

My first gift for the day is to offer my client, Darshana, some extra time during the phone session we have scheduled. Darshana, a women's health counselor, was my very first client many years ago, when I still worked full time at ad agencies. I consulted for Darshana on the side, helping her launch her company, Fruition Health. Since then I've had the joy of watching her business grow through many transitions.

These days, I consult on all areas of Darshana's business—marketing, operations, and management. Today we are supposed to talk about her plan to attract more clients who want to work over the phone because she recently moved to a little town outside of Santa Cruz, a much smaller market than San Francisco where she spent the last several years. She wants to counsel women all over the world, which means embracing new ways of working and communicating.

Over time, my relationship with Darsh evolved and we are now close friends. She has also been a health counselor to me for the past five years, supporting me through many changes in my life. Right after my MS diagnosis, Darsh helped me research the many different diets that are suggested for people diagnosed with MS and other autoimmune disorders. She was instrumental in helping make changes to the way I eat to help support my health—like giving up refined sugar and adjusting my fat intake to higher-quality fats that my body can metabolize better.

"I have exciting news," says Darsh at the beginning of our call.

"You bought a new house," I blurt excitedly. I know she and her husband have been home hunting for some time now.

"Nope," she says.

"You landed a new client."

"No, that's not it either. You'll never guess."

"Oh my God! You're pregnant!"

Darsh is silent.

"That's it, isn't it? You're going to have a baby!"

Darsh begins to laugh excitedly. I love the sound of her musical giggle.

"Oh my God. I'm so happy for you!"

"I can't believe it. We just started trying last month. We didn't think it would happen this fast."

I feel a little stab of envy. Darsh knows me well and reads my mind.

"I'm sorry, Cami," she says. "I know you and Mark have been trying to get pregnant for a long time. It must be hard to hear this news."

For the first year I was sick, Mark and I religiously had sex a few times around my ovulation time every month whether we felt like it or not. This scheduled baby-making sex quickly became mechanical and rather uninspiring for both of us. Month after month, I got my period, and we both felt more and more disappointed, making the distance between us grow. Darsh is one of the close friends I confided in each month during that time. *"Why aren't we getting pregnant?"* I wondered over and over again aloud to her. Mark and I even went in for fertility testing and were told nothing was wrong.

When my health started a more dramatic downhill slide, sex and a desire to get pregnant disappeared. What use would I be as a mother if I was too weak and sick to take care of a child? Even adoption really doesn't make sense these days unless my health turns around dramatically. It makes me sad to think I may miss out on the experience of motherhood. Adoption may be possible for us at some point, but right now, I have accepted that it just doesn't make good sense. In the meantime, I can be a terrific aunt to my niece and nephew and to the children of my friends.

"No, no," I insist. "I'm so happy for you. Sure, I hope it will happen for us, too, but I'm thrilled for you guys. You'll be an awesome mom. And Chris will be a fantastic dad."

"Chris is over the moon," she tells me.

"This is such great news. I can't wait to meet the baby."

"I suppose we should get down to business," says Darsh. "I don't want to pay you to gush about my pregnancy."

I tell Darsh not to worry about it, that I haven't started the clock for our business call yet. Then I offer her an extra thirty minutes for free.

She gratefully accepts and changes our planned agenda for the call a bit. In addition to marketing plans to bring in phone clients, she wants to figure out the best way to notify clients of her pregnancy and how to handle taking time off after the baby is born.

One hour later, we have ironed out solid ideas for all these issues. I hang up feeling satisfied that we made so much progress together and smile at the vision of Darsh with a pregnant belly. *I'm pretty sure she will have a little girl,* I think as I put her client file away.

I do another sink full of dishes as a little gift to Mark and then I give one more gift for the day. I take a canister of yummy Korean citron tea to my next door neighbor, Tyna. I don't know her well, but we've exchanged pleasantries on the balcony that we share.

"What is it?" Tyna asks as I hand her the jar of orange jelly-like substance.

I tell her that if she dissolves a tablespoon of the goo in hot water and takes a sip, she'll discover the most delicious tea she'll ever drink.

"I've heard that it's great mixed with vodka or sake," I tell her. "I don't drink, so haven't actually tried that."

"Hmm. We're having people over for a little party this weekend. Maybe we'll give it a try." Tyna has her long brown hair up in a ponytail and it bounces around as she talks.

She puts the jar into her refrigerator and we both sit down in her aqua 1950s-style dining chairs to talk. We discover that we're both voracious readers. During our discussion about the merits of "chick lit" versus the classics, we decide to begin a book swap. When we finish reading a book, we'll leave it on the table on our balcony so the other person can devour it next.

She sends me home with a little pile of novels, but I'm more excited about our budding friendship. Tyna and I have a lot in common. We both write. We both love animals. And we are both kind of introverted, warming up to new people slowly. Offering her a gift today helped break the ice that sometimes stands in the way of intimacy.

gift 29 ~ *Miracle Mile*

Today I give with enthusiasm is my affirmation for today, the
final day of my ritual. Mark and I have big plans to celebrate
the end of my giving cycle, but before we leave the house, I
want to donate some money to a cause or two. Ironically, giving money this month has helped relieve my financial inse-
curity. Even though we're still in debt, I now believe that we
have enough money—and, more important, that it is okay to
share what we have with others.

Someone recently posted a story on the Giving Challenge
website about giving a micro-loan to an entrepreneur in a
third-world country through Kiva.org. The loans are repaid
over time and then the money can be reloaned to other business owners in need. I want to do the same. I log on to the
Kiva site and search through the many people who are seek-
ing small amounts of cash. I choose to give a $25 loan to a
woman who runs a food market in Ghana. With a few clicks
of my mouse, the money is on its way across the world to
help her purchase a cart to assist in moving her produce. I
also write a check for $25 and mail the donation to the
FINCA Village Banking project, which helps women business owners in developing countries.

Mark and I both put on our running shoes and climb into
the car for what we're calling my Grand Finale: a 1-mile hike

at Runyon Canyon. We drive the short distance to the trail entrance. I grab my water bottle as we get out of the car and then set out on the trail, which quickly curves to the left and begins to slope upward. Though we've driven through the Hollywood Hills many times, this is my first time walking on one of the trails. I stop at the base of the gently sloping hill. Maybe I'm being too ambitious.

"That looks steep. I don't know if I can do this, honey," I tell Mark. "I think five or six blocks is the farthest I've walked so far. A mile might be pushing it."

"It's okay. We'll just go as far as you can. There's a bench right around the first curve so you can sit and rest up there," assures Mark. He has come up here running a few times. "If we make it all the way up to that peak and back down, it will be a little over one mile." He is pointing to an area that levels off where a number of people are gathered looking out over the canyon at what is likely a gorgeous view of L.A. on this clear day.

I take a deep breath. The sloping hill looks like Mount Everest to me.

"Okay. I'll try." I take Mark's hand and we begin our slow trek. Thankfully the trail is packed hard from the thousands of feet that have taken this walk before us. I wouldn't be able to keep my footing on top of loose dirt.

My legs are shaking by the time we reach the bench.

"My feet are tingling," I tell Mark. We sit down and Mark suggests that I take my shoes off for a bit.

"I don't think that's the best idea," I say to him. "The swelling always follows the tingling. If I take my sneakers off, I probably won't be able to get them back on."

"Do you want to go back down, then?" he asks. I can tell he's disappointed by the idea of turning around. So am I.

"No, no. Let's go. I can do it."

Mark smiles and offers his hand to me. I take hold and he gives me a helpful pull off the bench. We walk the remaining quarter mile, which curves back to the right and plateaus in an area with several benches. They are all full of people, most with dogs at their feet. One little Yorkie comes running up to me and throws himself down at my feet. He rolls over, belly up, reminding me of Habib when she begs for a good pet.

I bend over and begin to rub his tummy. The dog wriggles around on his back in pleasure until his owner calls him.

"Sampson, come."

At the sound of his mother's voice the little dog flips over and jumps to his feet. He runs down the trail and leaps up and down, begging his mom for affection. She leans down and obliges him, scratching behind his tiny ears.

"Maybe we should get a dog," I say to Mark as we snag a couple of newly vacated seats on a bench. I take a few chugs off my water bottle and admire the view of the HOLLYWOOD sign and the downtown L.A. skyline to my left. The mountains are visible beyond that. The city isn't cloaked in the heavy curtain of smog that normally obstructs the view from the Hollywood Hills. To my right, I can see all the way out to the coast, where the Pacific Ocean comes to kiss the shore in Santa Monica and Venice.

"Maybe we could see how we do taking care of a dog since we know a child isn't possible right now," I continue.

"I like that idea. I always wanted a dog when I was a kid,

but my parents wouldn't let us get one," says Mark. Then after a pause, "I can't believe this view."

"I know. It's because of the rain the other day. It cleaned out the air," I reply. I take Mark's hand. "We could get a small dog," I offer. "They're easier to take care of than big dogs."

"We'll have to talk to the landlord to see if she'll allow a dog in the apartment," Mark says, and then promises to speak with her.

The walk back down the hill is much easier than the climb up. Mark holds my hand the whole way down and we arrive back at the car triumphantly.

"I just walked a mile!" I exclaim to Mark, as if it were a marathon. To me it is.

"I know. And half of it was uphill," Mark says. He embraces me in a big sweaty hug, and we sway together in celebration.

We drive home and, as predicted, my feet swell up to grapefruits as soon as I remove my shoes. I prop them up on some pillows and rest for the remainder of the day. *I walked a mile today. I walked a mile today. I walked a mile today.* I repeat this phrase over and over again until the miracle sinks in.

Lying down nursing my swollen feet and legs, I reflect on the changes I've been experiencing. From the first day I started giving, the energy in my life changed direction. I felt that I wanted to be here, I deserved to be here. And I now believe on a deeper level that I am good enough.

I'm more capable of receiving assistance and love. In fact, I now enjoy reaching out my hand to offer or receive help.

It is easier for me to laugh and smile. Fun is easier to find.

I am more in awe of the people around me and tend to notice their good qualities rather than their "flaws."

I'm actually engaged in life again instead of just tolerating it. I'm showing up in the world in a different way, and that has dramatically improved my relationships—with my husband, with my parents, and now with old and new friends on the www.29Gifts.org website as they begin their 29 days of giving. It's just not possible to have positive interactions with people if your mind is stuck in a negative place.

Before, most of my energy and time had been going to a *lack,* to what I *wasn't* capable of: I wasn't earning much money anymore; Mark and I probably weren't going to be able to buy a house or have a baby. The path I'd been on was gone. Instead of staring down that empty path and bemoaning my fate, I began looking at little new paths that seemed to be magically unfolding in front of me. To my utter surprise, they took me away from that empty place and toward a new one I hadn't been able to imagine. I no longer feel a burning need to know exactly what is coming next in my life, nor do I feel the need to control everything anymore.

I am in significantly less physical and emotional pain. It's not that I got stronger overnight. The strength was there inside me the whole time—it just didn't feel worth it to come up with the energy I would need to claim it.

Perhaps the biggest change is that today I feel spiritually in touch with a higher sense of power. I have begun to see that *everything* belongs to the divine. God is in everything, including me. When we give or receive, we are connecting to that force. I now see I am a small part of a much greater whole, rather than the self-contained, deserted island I felt like 29 days ago. Today I see my interdependence with other people and with God as a source of power in my life. For most of my life I saw this sort of dependence as a liability and believed firmly that I must stand on my own two feet. I felt certain it was not wise to rely on anyone but myself. Breaking down that belief to acknowledge the presence of God and my need for other human beings in my life has left me with a new sense of freedom and independence of spirit.

In the wise words of Mahatma Gandhi, "The best way to find yourself is to lose yourself in the service of others." The past 29 days have proven this to be true for me.

I send out a prayer of gratitude to Mbali as my gift for the day. And I realize something I think I've known on some level practically since the beginning: Tomorrow I'm going to start all over again with Day 1.

Epilogue

ONE-YEAR CHECKUP

Today marks my 365th consecutive day of giving. I am in the midst of my thirteenth 29-day giving cycle. My life looks completely different today than it did one year ago.

I wish I could say that giving 29 Gifts cured my multiple sclerosis, but that would be dishonest. I still live with the effects of this disease, but the difference is that I cope a lot better. I now get through most days with only two prescription pills. I still inject myself daily with a drug that slows the progression of my MS, and it seems to be working, according to my doctors. In fact, my latest MRI scan shows there has been no new disease progression in the past year. Chronic pain is still a part of my life, and I sometimes take over-the-counter pain medication. Other than that, I take a few vitamin supplements and herbs to help support my immune system, and I try my best to eat well.

Though physical pain is still a constant in my life, it doesn't control me anymore. I'm able to work a little bit each day—usually about two hours. I am productive again and really enjoy the work I do.

Most days, I can walk on my own. I have had a few rough patches in the past year that required me to get a new cane. Once in a while—if I get overtired or push myself too much—I need the cane or an arm to hold on to when I walk. I no longer see this as a sign of weakness, but rather view my determination to continue walking as a source of strength. The distance I'm able to walk differs each day. Sometimes it is up and down my hallway at home. Other times, I'm able to go outside and walk anywhere between six and twelve blocks. When I'm not feeling my best, I still use the trick of walking laps around my block so I can stay close to home.

My relationships with my husband, family, and friends are more intimate and fulfilling. Mark and I get along better than ever. We still aren't parents but are again considering adopting a child. Mark and I are also discussing the possibility of becoming foster parents to provide shelter and stability to children who need it during times of family crisis.

In the meantime, we've added a dog to our family, an adorable little 5-pound Chihuahua named Charlie that we rescued from a bad living situation. Nursing Charlie back to health and rehabilitating him from a scared, shaky little dog into a confident, loving, sociable pooch has been rewarding for us. Charlie rarely leaves my side and I think of him as my baby.

Sadly, I recently lost my big, black cat Abu, who had been with me for fourteen years, since he was a tiny kitten. Habib is still healthy, but I miss Abu every day. Eventually we may get another kitten or a little dog to keep Charlie company.

My relationship with money has also changed dramatically. Though we still owe my father a large sum, we continue to make our payments to him each month. But I no longer worry about whether we have enough money. I've come to view money as an endless resource that exists in the world, and I trust that God will provide us with the funds to meet our needs.

Today I have a large community of friends in L.A. and I continue to stay close to my extended community of friends in San Francisco and the Midwest through regular phone calls and interaction online.

One of the biggest differences I see in my life today is that people tell me they love me several times a day and I tell them I love them, too. One year ago, I was in too much pain to allow love to be part of the picture.

I still cry sometimes when I have a hard day, but more often, I find myself tearing up because I'm overwhelmed with gratitude or moved by an amazing story from one of the givers on the 29 Gifts website.

Today, I'm part of a large group of people committed to the vision of a worldwide goodwill movement. Our collective mission is to create a grassroots revival of the giving spirit in the world. As of this writing, nearly 5,000 people in 38 countries have committed themselves to the 29-Day Giving Challenge by signing up on our website at www.29Gifts.org. More than 8,000 stories and 2,000 pieces of art have been posted.

Together as a community we have done some powerful work, proving that we can do together what we cannot do alone. We helped one of our fellow young 29Givers, Elysia Skye—who was recovering from breast cancer—raise more than $10,000 in only thirty days to help pay for a much-needed surgery. Most recently we helped Mbali raise nearly $5,000 to fund a humanitarian trip to South Africa with Vukani Mawethu, the choir she sings with, an award-winning, nonprofit multiracial choir that sings the freedom songs of South Africa and also gospel, spirituals, and civil rights songs linking people in the United States, South Africa, and around the world. During their South African tour, Mbali and the choir raised money for many worthy causes in her homeland and they had the distinctive honor of giving a private concert for Nelson Mandela.

I've found the new voice I yearned for during my first divination with Mbali, and I write almost every day now. When people ask me what I do, I always reply, "I'm a writer." I've even managed to write a whole book, with a lot of help from my friends!

I couldn't be more grateful to the people who have chosen to take part in the 29-Day Giving Challenge. I see our community as a place where we can all come to strip away the masks we tend to wear in our day-to-day lives. Most important, it's a place where we can all shine our collective light out into the world through the power of story and art.

Giving mindfully and being actively grateful for all I am receiving has become a part of my daily spiritual practice. Each day, I practice a simple series of actions that have developed into a formula for happiness that works for me without fail. This formula was suggested to me by Reverend Mark Vierra during a church service at the North Hollywood Church of Religious Science during my second cycle of giving:

God Consciousness + Giving + Gratitude = Abundance

Here's how this simple formula works. I pray and spend at least a few minutes in meditative reflection each day, I give at least one gift to another person whose path I'm blessed to cross. And I say thank you as many times as I can.

I have learned much about myself over the past 365 days. I've discovered that I am a good person at heart. I've learned that my value as a person isn't measured by how much I accomplish. I've embraced that I am so much more than the physical; the limitations multiple sclerosis imposes on my body do not stop me from living a purposeful life. I discovered that I have the power to touch other people and move them to action.

So today, on my 365th day of giving, I want to send out a sincere thank you to every person who has chosen to take part in the 29 Gifts Movement and to invite all of you to visit the site at www.29Gifts.org and sign up, too. And once again, I wish to express my deepest gratitude to Mbali Creazzo and the many other teachers who have passed on their wisdom and given me the inspiration to move forward with my life.

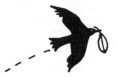

II

Stories from the
29 Gifts Community

The following true stories offer a snap-shot of the thousands of giving tales that can be found on the 29Gifts website. Visit www.29Gifts.org if you'd like to share a giving story of your own.

Icing on the Cake

Rudy Simone

I am standing in line waiting to check out at a Dollar Store. Few things here cost a dollar, but you do get some good deals. It's where I go when I am in a hurry, as I know where everything is and there are usually no more than one or two people in line. Today it's taking longer than usual to check out. I am passing the time by looking at the many pictures of Brad and Angelina that grace the covers of glossies I'd never open, though the longer I stand here the more tempting it gets. I am saved from temptation as the line moves forward. Only one customer ahead of me now.

"That will be $11.60," says the cashier in a bored, automated voice.

The lady in front of me digs through her wallet, trying not to drop her purse. She pushes her glasses back up on her nose as she counts change on a little ledge separating her from the cashier.

"Oh, I don't have enough money with me," she says apologetically. She is smiling, but you can see that she is squirming a little, embarrassed that her shortage of cash is on public display. Behind me I hear feet shuffling, audible exhales. The line is growing every moment and there's no other cash register open.

Rudy Simone is a writer living in Western New York.

"Do you have a card? We take debit and credit cards." The cashier's voice is unsweetened.

"No, I don't." She winces. "I'll have to put something back."

The cashier removes the items she'd placed into the bag, lays them a little roughly on the counter.

There's a box of birthday candles, a cake mix, a can of frosting, some candy, and some toys. The toys come in pairs. There are two packets of stickers, two bubble-blowers, two little girls' jewelry sets and two generic Barbie dolls.

"How much is this?" asks the customer, holding up the can of icing.

"$1.99."

It isn't enough to help the woman out of her plight. Something else will have to go. I can see her reluctance to choose. The cashier is showing signs of impatience: a slight edge in the tone of her voice, a slight downturn at the corners of her mouth, and a little line between her brows. Meanwhile, the line behind me is growing still longer. I stand there watching the cashier subtly but powerfully ruin this woman's day by trading that tiny little thing called compassion for contempt. The woman holds up a doll. I can't stand it.

"How much do you need?" I ask.

"What?"

"How short are you?"

The cashier raises an eyebrow and answers for her. "$2.60."

"Here." I hand her three dollars. I don't want to draw attention to myself, I don't want gratitude, and I don't want to hurry the lady up. I just want her to be happy, and I want both little girls to have a doll of her own to play with.

"Thank you so much," says the lady. "I have my two grand-daughters in the car. They're twins and today is their birthday. I thought I had more money with me."

"Don't mention it. Glad to help."

I really don't want thanks. This is one of the few times I have ever given something to someone without having some sort of self-interest. I donate clothes to charity all the time, but they're clothes I don't want anymore that are just taking up much-needed space in my closet. I give other things, too, but there's usually some thought of payback, even if it's karmic payback, behind my actions. And so it is for most of us most of the time. Sociologists, psychologists, philosophers, and theologians have always debated the concept of *altruism,* a term that was coined by Auguste Comte in the early 1800s. It means *something that is motivated purely by wanting to benefit another.* Dissenters say there is no such thing as true altruism; that no one's motives are ever entirely forgetful of self, since we know that we will feel good about ourselves and receive approval from others as a result of giving.

But for a moment I feel it in my heart. I want to help this woman, pure and simple. I want her to be happy and for her and the twins to have a pleasant day. Altruism exists. But, it too has a twin, one which is always close by. For immediately after that feeling, the thought enters my mind that I now feel pretty good about myself. But that is not my motivation, it is merely the icing on the cake.

Giving Lesson
Mary Woods

Note: Names in this story have been changed to protect privacy.

I work with kids every day who are current models of the bullies I remember from junior high. My fellow teachers and I are particularly challenged by one boy—I'll call him Bad Boy. He wears his jeans drooping precariously, an oversized, unwashed sweatshirt hanging down (thankfully) to cover the gap his pants leave, and ratty-looking sneakers. When he shoves his too-long hair out of his eyes, he reveals his sneering face. He looks like he doesn't have anybody clucking after him like mothers are supposed to.

Naturally, he's the bad-boy hottie of the sixth grade. He saunters slowly and deliberately, soaking up attention every step of the way. He's what teachers call a "negative leader," someone who is gifted with natural charisma but chooses to use it to pick on other kids, annoy the crap out of his teachers, and do as little actual work as possible. He's smart, but why bother?

Unfortunately, being a smart-ass turns people off, and that has happened to Bad Boy. His adoring audience of sighing girls remains faithful as ever, but I sense fellow teachers giving up on him. It showed up at Christmas. Teachers and staff at our school donate money to give kids who desperately need it for

---

Mary Woods is a middle school teacher and mother of two who lives in the Midwest.

Christmas. Wonderful, caring idea, right? During one of our meetings, we discussed who we thought needed some help—a sweet girl whose parents were living at the shelter; a recent immigrant who clearly only had one or two outfits; a hard-working girl with limited skills who had recently been placed in foster care. I thought about how Bad Boy wore the same clothes every day, about the distant look I'd seen on his face when he wasn't on stage in front of his peers.

"What about Bad Boy?" I tossed out. The rest of the teachers looked at me like I was crazy.

"I'm not sure I feel like he deserves this kind of a gift," someone replied.

"He certainly won't appreciate it; he won't be grateful," said another.

"All he's done all year is create trouble," said another, "So why should we reward that with a gift like this? What will that teach?"

I'm the softy in our group of teachers; I've been called "Pollyanna" for my optimistic attitude toward kids. To keep the peace, I let the topic of Bad Boy drop.

He was still on my mind that evening as I watched TV with my husband. I thought about the 29 Gifts movement, how we don't give to receive. It felt wrong to withhold this gift.

"I just don't think it's the right thing to do . . . I know he's a smart-ass and a punk, but . . ." Unexpectedly, my eyes welled up.

"He's a little boy," my husband finished. "At the heart of it, he's an 11-year-old boy. Somewhere in there, I hope, is a little boy who wants to get something for Christmas."

The next day after school, I talked to my principal, who agreed. I donated the money myself and it was given in a gift card. Nobody, including Bad Boy, would know who went to bat for him. I hope he wonders who actually gives a damn. Maybe he'll blow the $20.00 on God knows what, but I know I slept better after my principal and I worked out our super-secret giving scheme. There are times when being a person who was born onto this Earth ought to be enough to "deserve" receiving a gift.

Reading Allowed

Steve Gentile

It is a slow time of year during my first 29-day cycle of giving. Time seems almost to have come to a halt. Folks take vacations, get ready to shuttle older kids to college, and the younger ones ready themselves for school. Feeling aimless, I find myself today in the town library, where my mother and I often visited when I was young. My phone won't ring, I won't be tempted to send or read e-mails, which are few and far between anyway. In the few hours I plan to spend here, I don't think I'll miss many developments in the outside world.

I go inside empty-handed, like I did so many times as a kid. I find the first classic book that comes to mind—Jack London's *Call of the Wild*—and search for a spot to read. Settling into a quiet corner near a window, I am soon joined by a small group of children having just the same plan, it seems. The four of them whisper like kids do (which isn't whispering at all), form a small circle, and start reading their shared book aloud.

It is *Charlotte's Web* by E. B. White. *A great choice,* I muse, resigned to the loss of peace and quiet. Each child takes a turn reading a few paragraphs, shows a picture if available, and passes it to their neighbor to continue. I stop reading my book, finding myself pleasantly distracted, oddly attracted to this simple activity. When I move to face them, they grow timid.

Steve Gentile shares his East Coast home with his wife and their two Airedale Terriers.

"Sorry, sir," one says.

"No need for that. Please read on."

They do. I listen peacefully. Each child in the circle reads as quietly as possible. Each helps with words another can't pronounce, doesn't understand, or has difficulty breaking down.

Their first inclination is to turn to me and ask for help with their eyes or voices. I guess it's because I am the closest adult.

"Some words are tough, keep trying," I encourage them.

It is a wonderful experience in so many ways. Without kids of my own, I have missed out on this simple pleasure. The sound of young voices trying newfound words on for size is priceless—the hesitation before an unknown word, the upturn of the voice when pronouncing it, as if to ask, "*Is that right?*" It's a gift to be treasured.

Listening to their young voices, I am once again a kid myself, but at the same time, I am my mother hearing me read aloud. Their words are in my head, in my mouth, and suddenly in the air around me. The moment is so delicious, present, and abundant, it seems never ending.

I realize my gift to them is rich. In allowing these children to continue without feeling as if they are imposing, and in listening to them completely, they are free to read fearlessly, to show off their command of the language. Somehow, through some small miracle, we all hold that sacred space.

Just as mysteriously as it all began, it ends. My young readers disperse. The world around us goes back to what it is. Clocks begin to measure time again. Life goes on, inside and outside the library—as real as the memory of the woman who brought me into this world loving words and language, my mom.

Thank you kids, for your gift of this quiet memory.

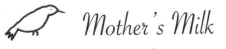

Mother's Milk

Erin Monahan

Pregnant women are "expectant mothers" because pregnancy carries the inherent promise of motherhood. We *expect* dirty diapers and sleepless nights, first steps and scraped knees, tears and giggles, nightmares and dreams. We do not expect to tuck our sweet baby into a 24-inch ivory casket. It's against the rules. Unfortunately, sometimes the universe changes all the rules. That is what happened to me, twice.

In a five-year span, my daughter, Alexis, and my son, Donovan (Nova), were each born with a life-threatening congenital heart defect. Twice, a language of medical terminology that I could barely pronounce defined my life. Twice, I begged and bargained with doctors and deities for the life of my child. Twice, I have selected a casket and watched cemetery workers cover it with dirt.

Alexis lived just twelve days. Her five big brothers and sister met her only once. They pressed their noses to the side of a plastic bassinette in the neonatal intensive care unit and said hello to their beautiful pink-cheeked baby sister when she was four days old. I remember her twelve-day life as a blur—a mix of pride, fear, love, and pain. She seemed fine for thirty-six hours. After that, we shared her with doctors, nurses, and surgeons. They fed her, changed her, held her, and rocked her to sleep far

Erin Monahan is a published poet and mother of five living in Indian Trail, North Carolina.

more often than I did. All I have left of her is a few pictures, a pink blanket, and a lock of her hair, all kept in a memory box tied with a jade-green ribbon.

I spent the next five years in a haze of fear, mistrust, and resentment. I was not a mother, a wife, a daughter, an employee, or a friend. I was a grieving woman and that was all I could manage. The world moved on, but the best I could do was go along for the ride. I felt nothing, except when I felt angry.

Then Nova was born. His heart defect, diagnosed in utero, was nearly identical to Alexis's, though slightly less severe. He was born in December, and we got to take him home for Christmas, where he stayed until he was three months old. To others, he appeared to be a healthy baby boy without a care in the world. For us, there were endless appointments, painful procedures, and countless sleepless nights, but even in the shadow of the inevitable open-heart surgery, we believed. The universe couldn't be cruel enough to break the rules again. However, on April 6, 2006, after six weeks of surgeries, complications, and infections, Nova succumbed to a fungal infection and died in my arms.

Our experience with Nova's life was far different from what we went through with Alexis. Instead of closing up on ourselves, we opened up to the world. We joined the American Heart Association. We talked to other parents in the same situation. I did television and newspaper interviews and addressed an audience of over 7,000. While we had held Alexis inside us as our private source of misery, we held Nova up as a light to illuminate the world. Nova reminded us to live, and he was the star that guided us to acceptance.

It has been a long journey to this "new normal" which is so unlike the "normal" I knew before. I am far more compassionate and entirely more generous because I have learned one key thing: Generosity lifts you up; it gives you a reason to feel good, even when you can no longer imagine what good feels like. When I found the 29-Day Giving Challenge, it struck me how perfectly it lent itself to my beliefs, and I joined with a sense of excitement. However, when it came time to give something I felt I would never part with, I discovered why this ritual is a challenge.

The only material thing I have ever become emotionally attached to was the breast pump I used for Alexis and Nova. Breast milk is better for all babies, but babies with heart defects have compromised immune systems, and the antibodies in breast milk help them fight infection. Since my babies were hospitalized early, they wouldn't latch onto my breast, so pumping my milk was the only thing I could do to help my babies stay strong and healthy. Although I couldn't save them, the breast pump came to symbolize my love for the babies I lost.

When Nova died, I was left with tons of baby stuff. The crib, the car seat, swing, bouncy seat . . . and the breast pump. I put it all in storage, but eventually everything was given away or loaned out. When my niece got pregnant and asked to borrow Nova's things—including the breast pump—I was reluctant, fearful that it wouldn't be returned. Thankfully, my concern was unfounded, and as a result, I loaned it to several other women over the next year or so.

Recently, someone with whom I attended elementary, middle, and high school, but hadn't seen in nearly twenty years, came back into my life. He and his girlfriend are pregnant and in financial dire straits. She wants to breastfeed, needs a breast pump, and of course, I have one I could gift her. I actually feel that I am supposed to let her use it, yet, I don't trust her to properly care for it or return it. I have spent weeks now vacillating with what to do.

When I feel led to do something, I usually answer the calling without hesitation. However, my mind swings back and forth between *Do it!* and *What if she breaks it? What if she never returns it?* I first decide to sell it to her, but she can't afford to buy it. I finally decide *not* to let her use it and even post the pump for sale on a local website and, later, at a yard sale, but no buyer comes.

Ever heard the phrase, "Never lend money that you can't afford to give away?" Basically, it means that if you lend money to anyone, don't do it until you have reconciled yourself with never getting repaid. That is how I choose to approach this. I am giving the breast pump to her now with no true expectation of getting it back. In essence, I am letting it go. I have reconciled myself to never getting this pump back, and accepted that The Universe wants it to go to this particular person. I gift it knowing that I have done exactly what I *should* do with it, and that Nova and Alexis are smiling down with approval.

A Different Way to Keep Warm

Jennifer Meriposa Fuller

The wind whipped around me, a biting chill making its way through my clothes. It seemed that the sunny Portland, Oregon, summer had given way immediately to winter, with no mild autumn in between. The weather had caught me off guard and I wasn't dressed for it, with only a thin sweater and jeans. To make matters worse, I had been talking to my friend for an hour on my cell phone while sitting in the park, meaning that my right hand now was a frozen claw. "Hot chocolate!" I exclaimed excitedly to myself. That was exactly what I needed. I made my way to the nearest corner coffee shop and ordered a medium cocoa. Usually I would get the large, but money was extremely tight for me these days, being unemployed for almost a year, and buying this hot chocolate at all was a treat.

I emerged from the coffee shop with that enormous satisfaction you feel when you've just received the exact thing you had been craving. I crossed the street, wind howling at me from all directions. And just as I was about to take that first glorious sip, I spotted a woman to my left. She was homeless, sitting on the cold concrete holding a cardboard sign. The woman was bundled as best as she could against the weather, but I imagined she must be freezing. Without thinking, I immediately walked

Jennifer Meriposa Fuller is happy to call Portland, Oregon, home.

over to her. "Would you like some hot chocolate?" I asked, and held out the cup.

The pained expression on her face changed in an instant. Her eyes got wide and bright with surprise and anticipation, like a kid at Christmas. The excitement on her face was a million times more than the satisfaction I was feeling seconds before. "Oh yes, thank you!" she chirped at me. I gave it to her with a huge smile on my face and continued down the street. As I walked away, she buried her face in the steam and reveled in its warmth.

Suddenly, I wasn't so cold anymore. It was as if the giving of something so small and simple, yet completely delightfully received, had literally warmed my soul. And to top it off, I couldn't stop smiling. Immediately I wanted to do more, as if I wanted to spread the contagiousness of happiness around. I walked down the street looking for others to help. It was an eagerness that was almost obsessive, probably visible. The giving had just felt so good.

Then it hit me. I hadn't thought twice about giving her that hot chocolate, even though I had been craving it for myself for about an hour. The moment I saw the woman, I just knew that she needed it far more than I did, and I automatically handed it over. I realized then that as I had been giving each day in the spirit of 29 Gifts, it had become second nature. I am so grateful that I get to experience the world around me in a different light, one that involves not only noticing others' desires but knowing that I have the ability to help fulfill them if I so choose. And that is a powerful thing.

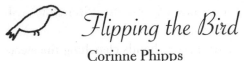
Flipping the Bird

Corinne Phipps

One fine April day in California, when I am driving home from the hair salon in my sturdy green Volvo, I have a close call.

Killer tunes are blasting on the radio. I am minding the traffic and my own business in the far right lane of a three-lane thoroughfare. It is a heavy traffic day, which makes little sense for this Silicon Valley town. *Maybe there is an accident up ahead,* I think. In 15 minutes I haven't even gone three blocks. But I am not particularly bothered with this—I have a cute new haircut and I am feeling pretty fly. And I'm thinking about my commitment to the 29-Day Giving Challenge.

What would be really cool to give away today? I wonder. Yesterday, I gave my favorite chocolates away to my chiropractor (I am still not sure what possessed me to do that). She was very appreciative, especially because she is four months pregnant.

All of a sudden, this blue Cabriolet guns it and starts changing lanes, right into *my* lane, cutting me off. I always leave a car length of space in front and behind me so I have time to slam on my brakes, but my heart begins beating in my throat. I have a hot temper and very little patience for bad drivers. As I slow down, it's all I can do to swerve to the right to miss the Cabriolet. Thank God my reflexes are quick—I barely have any room, or time, to move to the shoulder. And thank goodness no one

Corinne Phipps is the founder of Urban Darling, a wardrobe styling company, and lives in Silicon Valley, California.

was walking down the sidewalk next to the shoulder. Now I'm freaking out, the kind of freakout where the adrenaline rush makes you feel like you are going to vomit.

While my heart is racing, sweaty hands clenching the steering wheel, the Cabriolet realizes its mistake and swerves back to the left, correcting its lane change.

Mother F—ker, can't they see that I am here? What an a—hole!!! These are my first thoughts as I stop seeing red. At this point, I would normally begin to wail on the horn, roll down the window, and call out all kinds of expletives, basking in my glory of being in the right. A good native San Franciscan knows how to drive. I catch my breath, take my hand off the window button and pause enough for reason to come in.

In this moment I remember my commitment to the 29-Day Giving Challenge. I take a few deep breaths and begin to calm down, but I have no idea that what I'm about to do will set me on a new course. The blue Cabriolet and I are neck and neck, stopped at the next light. I look over at the driver, irritated. The driver, a guy, waves and mouths, *"Sorry."*

Once upon a time, I would have flipped him one middle finger, commonly referred to as "The Bird." Instead, two fingers pop up, and I throw him the peace sign. I begin to giggle. When the light turns green, I smile and wave. Now this is something that I have never done before—forgiving a driver for a misjudgment! I am in shock. I feel better about myself, that now I have made a very small difference in his life, and my own. I feel like I float home in my car.

That is what I gave that day in April. Once it would have been The Bird, but today it was forgiveness, compassion and, best of all, Peace.

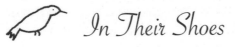

In Their Shoes

Pamela Rosin

It had been my dream for many years to visit India, so when my friend Juliana said, "Come with me!" I jumped at the chance. I wanted to drink in the beauty and the chaos, to breathe in the air of a culture and spirituality with a depth of history far greater than my own. More than anything, I wanted to expand my sense of the world through contact with a place so starkly in contrast with what I knew.

During the last part of my visit I traveled alone and hired a driver, quite a luxurious way to see the country. It meant I could cover a lot of ground, staying in a total of thirteen cities by the month's end. Seated in this comfy, air-conditioned car, I was overwhelmed by the life I saw through the windows. I zipped past scenes of unfathomable poverty and utter destitution. I saw a man with no legs maneuver himself across the street on his hands; I remember gasping as the throng of traffic narrowly missed hitting him. I saw mountains of trash. I saw entire families riding a single moped. And I saw an innovation and creativity to make do with so little.

I realized how much time I'd spent on the trip feeling apprehensive and thinking about my own needs—hunger, having to pee, heat, exhaustion, thirst! From behind the glass I felt acutely aware of my privilege and wanted some contact with the

---

Pamela Rosin lives in San Francisco.

people. It got me thinking, what could I possibly do? What could I do that would have an impact at all?

Through talking with Mohan, my driver, I came up with the idea of shoes. I could give flip-flops and sandals to children primarily, as well as to adults. Mohan agreed to help me and it became our pet project. When we arrived in the next town, Tanjavor, we weaved on foot through the night market and the bustle of Divali (a Hindu festival) shoppers to reach a shoe vendor, who sold me seventy pairs of sandals. I also bought forty notebooks and as many pens to give away. The bustling market occupied eight blocks in each direction. The city streets were filled with vendors and people of all ages, even young children.

I felt so alive that night. I was in the crowds but didn't mind the stares. I was energized by my project, thrilled by the enormous bag of shoes carried back to Mohan's car by a young man on his bicycle.

The next morning I was filled with anticipation about giving away the shoes. But soon I discovered what a complex thing giving can be.

For my first attempt, I was invited into a home where beautiful silk saris are made. I was led upstairs to the two rooms, where the teenage son and daughter each sat at a loom that took up almost the entire room. Their legs were just long enough to reach the pedals of the loom. I bought a couple of lovely iridescent silk scarves.

As I was ready to leave, I asked the father if I could give his children sandals. But within minutes the entire neighborhood had assembled with an eagerness to partake in the shoe giveaway. After clumsily sorting through shoes and trying to find ones that fit for the rambunctious crowd that had gathered, Mohan soon gave up and whisked me and the shoes away. It was an awful scene; when he pulled us away, some of the children were in tears. I felt terrible, and yet reluctantly I could see Mohan's point. To avoid mayhem, we would have to be strategic about it. We would only stop where a few children were gathered along the road.

Later, he gave me a few pairs of shoes to keep in the back seat for our drive-by gifting. The reactions to the shoes were mixed. After many plastic bags landed on the ground unclaimed, I decided to unwrap the sandals first. But Mohan explained that people assume the shoes are used and are not interested in them. Sometimes I would offer shoes to older women and realized they'd probably never worn shoes in their lives. Sometimes I got a blank stare; I wasn't sure if I'd offended people. Sometimes they'd ask what else I had or whether I had more for family members. Once after I gave sandals to a pair of brothers, I looked back as we pulled away to see the younger one dance a jig of celebration. Once as the road rounded a bend between rice paddies, we passed a little girl of about 9 in a blue school uniform on a bicycle. I rolled down the window, asked her if she wanted some sandals, and dropped them into the basket of her bike, right on top of her books. Her face lit up with the most beautiful smile.

Sometimes when you open up to give, you must really let in the pain of others' suffering. It doesn't always flow easily and abundantly. I discovered I had to let go of my preconceived notion of how my gift would be received as well as how I would feel as I gave. I had to let go of my attachment to the recipients' reactions. I think my idealized fantasy of giving was born from that comfy, isolated place behind the car window, where I wanted to have an impact. Being in the moment and letting the people react to my gift, or even refuse it, humbled me and let their reality touch me in a deep way. Kind of like stepping into their shoes.

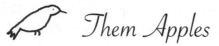

Them Apples

Whitney Ferrall

It all started with the apples. Granny Smith, Pink Lady, Fuji, Arkansas Black.

On the drive back from Hilltop Orchard, I survey our over-flowing baskets and imagine what we might do with all those apples. A bushel and a half. That's how many we have.

By the time we pull up to the house, I have plans to make crisps, sauce, butter, dried rings, and pie. I will drop off a crisp with a pregnant friend, and take jars of apple butter to the neighbors.

After joining the 29-Day Giving Challenge, I am determined to make good on all of those nice thoughts. The meals promised to pregnant friends, the care-packages sent to loved ones far away. I have always been quick to offer such things, but slow to deliver. This time is no different. Something always seems to distract me. The kids, a phone call, an impromptu visitor. The apples sit.

One day I finally get so far as to mix the oats, flour and butter for a breakfast crisp. My in-laws are staying with us for the weekend and I think it might be nice to wake up with a little crisp and coffee. I am just about to peel my first apple when my husband enters. His parents want to go out to breakfast. We

---

Whitney Ferrall is a daughter, writer, sister, wife, mother, volunteer, artist and friend. She lives in Charlotte, North Carolina.

stay busy all weekend, and on Monday the real madness begins, and I never get back to the crisp. The apples sit.

In the meantime, I offer smiles to strangers, make a few small donations, and give many gifts of time. According to the 29 Gifts rules of giving, all of these efforts count as long as they are done with thought and purpose, but none of them seem as grand as homemade apple treats.

Perhaps I was inspired by my high school efforts at purposeful giving, which began junior year when my Leadership classmates and I participated in Random Acts of Kindness Week. The most popular random act of kindness was to treat the next customer in the drive-through to a cookie. Where a smile or kind word might be disregarded, food always seemed to get a warm reception.

On Day 8, the phone rings. It's Mary, a mom-friend. "I'd like to come over today, if that's okay," she says. "Tom's out of town and I really need to get out of the house."

It isn't okay, really. I want to be alone, as alone as I can be, anyway, with two young children in the house. I have big plans to stick the kids in front of a video and catch up on some computer work. I don't even know Mary that well—doesn't she have a real friend she could call? Maybe not. I think of her, very pregnant and trying to keep up with a two year old, and I know that she needs company more than I need time alone.

"Sure," I say. "Come on over."

When I'm on a deadline, my usual routine of working late at night and two mornings a week doesn't cut it. I have to infringe on my parenting hours, which basically means staring at the computer much of the day while the children play around me. This is hardly efficient. My toddler regularly climbs into my lap for a book or a snack, my three year old pauses to share a story, the two fight over a toy or make a mess that needs immediate attention. Still, I manage to make a dent in the project, and that keeps me in the circus. I'm sorry to lose that time today, but I look forward to tomorrow, when I'll be able to put in a few hours writing at the coffee shop while both kids are in preschool.

The next morning, I pack up my laptop along with the kids' lunches, eager to have a few hours at the coffee shop while they are in preschool.

And then: an emergency. Two teachers are out sick, there aren't enough subs, and it's Picture Day. I only signed up as co-chair for picture day because it was advertised to be an easy gig; a little e-mailing, a few phone calls, *no* on-site volunteering. "You're staying, aren't you?" Ms. Cathie, the director of the preschool, looks to me expectantly. She's not really asking. *No, I'm not staying,* I want to say. *Just because I don't go to an office doesn't mean I'm not working. I have deadlines. I have people depending on me.* I've been dealing with the misconception a lot lately, that freelancing isn't really working, and I'm feeling a little bitter about it. It takes considerable patience not to go off on Ms. Cathie.

I think of the 29-Day Giving Challenge. Time will be my gift today. "Of course," I answer. "Where do you need me?"

I spend the next four hours outside, wiping crusty noses and combing hair so that each child sparkles for the candid photos. This is my turning point in the challenge.

I am beginning to realize that my time is as great a gift as any other, that it may be better, even, than apples. When the school day ends, I drive home, return my unused laptop to the desk, and sit on the floor to play with the kids.

Later on, I do try to squeeze some work into the afternoon,

but when my daughter comes to me with another seemingly endless story of gibberish, I make an effort to look at her when she talks, instead of continuing to stare at the computer screen and offer only an occasional nod and an "uh-huh."

My goal is to be more conscious in the moment, whatever I am doing, whoever I am with. With each day's gift, I strive to focus on my children, my husband, my friends, the mom in a bind, the stranger next to me in line, to give them all of myself, if only for a bit, before moving on to the next task that must be done. The gift of time may not be as heart-warming as apple pie, but it is at least as powerful.

Turns out that Mary, the lonely mom who invited herself over, doesn't have many friends in town. She had moved from out of state in the middle of her second pregnancy, and all the unpacking and resettling didn't allow her to get out much. The afternoon we spent together was restorative for both of us, and I am grateful to have found this new friend. I think I'll take over some apples when she has the baby. Not a crisp, or a tart, or a pie. Instead of spending that time in the kitchen, I'll hand-deliver some plain old apples—a nice mix of Granny Smith, Pink Lady, Fuji and Arkansas Black—and then we'll spend that time together.

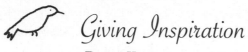

Giving Inspiration

Daryn Kagan

I should've known. I should've remembered. And yet, it is the lesson I get the joy of relearning over and over again.

The lesson? That the Universe conspires to make it easy for me to give *and* rewards me many times over with gifts way beyond anything I can imagine.

My lesson starts with losing my job. Odd to start a story about giving with losing something. And yet, it often takes loss to get us on a better track.

I had a dream television news job anchoring news for CNN. I was there for 12 years, covering everything from war to the red carpet of the Oscars. I had the privilege of anchoring some of the most important breaking stories of my lifetime, like the events of September 11, 2001. Basically, if you love doing news, this was the place to do it.

Why don't we grab a coffee after you get off the air, the e-mail from the big boss read that fateful day.

Honestly, I thought he was calling me in to tell me what a great job I had done at the anchor desk that day. I was wrong.

"I know your contract is up at the end of the year," Big Boss started, "and I just wanted you to know that we won't be renewing with you."

Daryn Kagan lives in Atlanta, Georgia, and is the author of *What's Possible! 50 True Stories of People Who Dared to Dream They Could Make a Difference.*

"Really?" I say. I am in shock, although after so many years in the news business, I shouldn't be.

I never did ask him why, but did eventually ask myself, "What?" As in, "What am I going to do now?" The question didn't come right away. First, I gave myself some time and space to have my sad; to grieve my dream job going away. Then, surprisingly, I decided that I no longer wanted to do TV news. It had been great, but I knew I was done.

I asked myself, *"If I could do anything I wanted, how could I serve the world?"*

The answer came straight from my heart. Tell inspirational stories. Serve as a vehicle to let those who inspire others to make a difference in the world.

The idea might make you feel all warm and fuzzy on the inside, but it was hardly what you might call the most practical. The old adage in the news business is that "If it bleeds, it leads." In other words, good news doesn't sell.

Also, I had no experience running my own company, and yet here I was, about to step out in that direction. To say I knew nothing about where I was headed would be giving me way too much credit. And yet, there was that lesson: Be optimistic, commit to giving, and the Universe will support you. I could fill a book with all the amazing turns of events and angels that have come my way.

There is one story in particular that happened early on that illustrates the above.

One of the first things you do when launching a web-based business is register your domain name. It's really no big deal. You just go to one of any number of websites, type in the URL, and click "Buy." The whole thing takes about a minute and costs less than $10.

So, off I went in mid-2006 to register DarynKagan.com. Much to my surprise, however, the screen refreshed only to tell me, "DarynKagan.com is taken."

"*Taken?*" I wondered aloud. "How can that be? There can't be a lot of Daryn Kagans running around."

I honestly thought all I had to do was call the company and have a little chat. I figured they would see the mistake and just give me my own name back. I was wrong.

"Lady, you have a problem," the voice on the other end of the line told me. "It's called 'cybersquatting.' It's totally legal. People grab names that they think someone will want and hope to make a lot of money selling them later. Get ready to pay tens of thousands, even hundreds of thousands of dollars. Or hire a really expensive lawyer."

"Well, shoot," I thought. "That's not how I wanted to start this new venture." I then decided to test the karma on this idea of giving inspiring stories to the world. I wrote the man who owned my name an e-mail.

His name was Thomas Boone and this is what my e-mail said:

Dear Mr. Boone,

    Thank you for thinking of me when you went to register domain names. But now I believe the time has come for DarynKagan.com to go back to its rightful owner, which of course, would be me. I spoke with the company and technically, it's no big deal. Three clicks and you can transfer ownership back to me.

    Sincerely,
    Daryn Kagan

I didn't mention money or lawyers.

This all led to a very interesting phone call the next day. Mr. Boone informed me he was a big fan of mine. He said he watched me all the time on CNN.

"Why do you think I have your name?" he wanted to know.

This made me a touch nervous. Was I talking to a stalker?

After I told Mr. Boone that I didn't have any idea why he had my name, he informed me that he had just figured it out. "I think I was meant to have it, and hold onto it," he explained, "so that no one would take advantage of you."

"Well, can I have it back now?" I asked in my sweetest of voices.

"Sure," he replied.

And by that night, I was indeed the rightful owner of DarynKagan.com. Not a dime changed hands and no, he didn't turn out to be some weird stalker. I think I heard from him once or twice in the following two years.

This type of thing has happened again and again, making it possible for me to share inspiring stories with people all around the world.

I first met Cami Walker while I was speaking at a women's business conference. She came up to me after my speech and briefly told me the 29 Gifts story. Her story touched me more than most. I decided that I, too, wanted to have the 29 Gifts experience. I signed up and started giving my gifts not long after meeting her.

The first gift I sent was a $15 Starbucks gift card to my little sister in New York City. It was kind of a silly gift to send, as she and her girlfriend owned their own coffee house at the time. But, in some way, it was perfect. My sister was thrilled. She might have been making a lot of coffee for others, but she rarely took the time to step away and give herself a coffee break. I also gave many anonymous gifts over the 29 days. Gas prices were sky high in the summer of 2008. One day I stopped in a station's mini mart. After paying at the pump, I took the time to go inside to the cashier. I handed over $10 and asked her to apply it to the next customer who came in. I got a double thrill out of that gift, as I pictured the stranger who would receive the ten bucks' worth of gas and the thrill the cashier would get by now being the giver.

During my 29-day giving experience, of course there was the daily glow that comes with giving, but there were also daily lessons. Just as Cami had suggested, I watched what I was giving. What was easy to give? What was hardest? 29 Gifts predicted that the thing that would be the most difficult to give would be the thing that felt the most scarce in my life.

As it turned out, my easiest thing to give was money. The hardest to give was a piece of myself; my heart. Emotional connections took more effort, like the day I gifted my mother with a phone call and photo in the middle of my water skiing vacation. I had to put aside some resentment. I recall thinking, *I'm way too old to have to check in with my mommy while I'm on vacation.* Instead, I saw it as the gift it was. Indeed, she loved hearing from me and seeing the beautiful Minnesota lake where I was visiting.

To borrow from my old career, the idea that giving leads to big-time getting is not breaking news to those who give. When you focus on others, more gifts than you could ever imagine end up coming back to you.

And each time I forget that, a lesson is lurking right around the corner to remind me.

A Letter from Mbali Creazzo

In the following letter to readers of this book, Mbali Creazzo shares the history of the 29-day giving ritual that inspired this project. She also offers a number of helpful tips and suggestions to assist you in getting the most out of your own 29-Day Giving Challenge, should you choose to commit to the exercise.

Dear Reader,

Sawubona, as the Zulus say in greeting.

The 29-Day Giving Challenge originated as an African ritual, but it's perfect for people living in the Western world. Giving of any kind—even a simple action—begins the process of change, and moves us to remember that we are part of a much greater universe.

The ritual of giving 29 gifts in 29 days came to me when my life was in a place of scarcity. I had been laid off from a job of eight years that I loved, and I feared I would lose everything. This 29-day giving ritual was prescribed by a healer in a Divination similar to those I perform for my students today. This method of Divination is a type of intuitive reading, using tools such as shells, bones, or stones to help people navigate their present situation based on information received from their ancestors.

In my work as a healer, I draw from the Dagara African tradition, first introduced to me by Malidoma Patrice Some, an edu-

The South African Medicine Woman who inspired the 29 Gifts Movement

cator and shaman who has written many books and speaks all over the world. Like many practices of a spiritual nature, my work is often subject to skepticism. It takes a special kind of faith and willingness to pursue healing through such nontraditional methods. For some, like Cami, it is desperation and frustration with a lack of progress through "traditional" means that brings people to my doorstep. I do not claim to offer "cures," and would never suggest a person abandon treatment by qualified medical professionals, but rather add any alternative healing techniques that resonate with them to complement their healing.

When I went to one of my teachers for a Divination during a challenging time in my own life, I remember feeling that to give at this time seemed more an act of recklessness on my part than kindness to others. I also recall feeling fearful about "giving up" what little I believed I had to call my own. But as a risk taker, I decided to embrace the 29-day giving ritual with an open heart.

I would like to relate just one of my giving experiences from my own 29-day giving ritual. During my Divination, my teacher told me that one of my gifts should be to a homeless woman on the street. My teacher said I would know the woman when I saw her. I had to give her a specific sum of money and buy her a meal. This may sound familiar to you from Cami's story in this book.

I carried the specific sum of cash in the car, and one evening I finally saw the woman I thought was "the one" after scanning the streets every day for a week. I was on my way home at midnight after a long, stressful day working in a homeless shelter. I felt I had given more than enough during my shift at work, and frankly, I felt resentful about having to give more that night. I could have easily gone home to my warm bed, but something told me to see this through.

It took me a while to find a place that served food that was still open. After I picked up the meal, I drove back hoping the woman would still be in the same spot. Of course, she wasn't. She had walked some distance, but I drove until I found her.

When I handed the food and wad of dollar bills to this woman, something profound happened for me. I was overwhelmed with humility and felt very comforted and peaceful. I also felt a rush of energy that refueled my spirit that, less than one hour ago, felt drained. I was curious as to why I felt so good afterward. Giving that night felt like a gift to me. When I reflected on it later, I came to this realization: When I am in service to another person, I am moving from a place of self-centeredness to selflessness. The act of giving inherently carries gratitude in it. For me, it is impossible to give without feeling grateful.

When that woman took her meal and money from my hand, I realized how much I did have. Just a week earlier, I was in a deep place of scarcity. I now felt instantly abundant. I did not have to walk the streets or sleep in the cold with nowhere to shower. I was not hungry, nor did I have to beg for money every day to survive. Last week, I was feeling lost, scared, angry, and sorry for myself, yet offering this simple gift made me feel so much more alive. I remember going home that night and getting on my knees to give thanks. Then I reflected on the genius of the diviner in her "prescription." I'm sure she knew that to connect with a homeless person on the street at this time would remind me of how much I still had and jostle me out of my self-pity.

That night, I chose to take my medicine by offering that gift. Not only did I feel better, but my life changed as a result. I left the job I was sad to lose and began to focus more on my healing practice. I began to pursue my goals of becoming an HIV/AIDS educator and counselor. It was not long after this that I began doing healing work with Cami.

After the night I offered my gift to the woman on the street, I took the following nine lessons with me:

1. When I give with an open heart, I receive the profound gift of humility.

2. Gratitude keeps my heart open.

3. Giving opens space for me to receive because giving and receiving are part of the same naturally reciprocal cycle.

4. Selflessness does not mean giving of myself to the extent that I am left depleted.

5. When I give from a place of service, honesty, and fullness, I am left feeling revitalized.

6. When I give from a place of responsibility and resentment, I negate the give and nothing changes. In fact, I'm often left feeling resentful and drained.

7. When I am immersed in self-centeredness as opposed to self-love, I become isolated and lonely and I forget I am part of a greater whole. The last thing I want to do is give.

8. When I give, I am living the practice of being truly human. When I practice making mindful connections with others, my life *feels* meaningful, therefore it is.

9. I rarely move back into a place of scarcity when I remember to give mindfully each day.

I believe the 29-Day Giving Challenge is fitting for the Western world because a scarcity mindset is common to many of us, no matter how much we have materially. Though most of us have no experience of the depth of scarcity that exists in

African countries, we often believe we are not successful enough, rich enough, beautiful or thin enough. We simply *don't have enough* or are *not good enough*. We become so lost in our *sense of lack, low self-esteem,* and *nonexistent self-love,* that we forget that our life is an essential part of a greater whole, and that we have many gifts to offer to the world at large.

I passed on this giving prescription to Cami out of fierce compassion and deep concern for her higher good. She could have chosen to take offense and stay stuck or accept the challenge and take action. She had the courage to choose the latter. I hope you will as well.

I hope you commit to your own 29-Day Giving Challenge and enjoy your journey. You can also use the online journal provided free at www.29Gifts.org to keep a record of your experience. As you begin, I invite you to turn your giving into a sacred ritual. Bring mindfulness to your daily giving practice and your journaling, so it becomes a transformative experience you will want to remember and refer back to.

In addition to journaling each day about the gift you offered, I suggest you also take time over your 29 days to reflect and write about the following:

- **Gratitude:** Note at least three things you feel grateful for each day. This may be anything from a family member, your health, shelter, or nature.
- **Lineage:** Over your 29 Days, take time to reflect on the tradition and history of giving in your family. What lessons did you learn from your parents, grandparents, or other ancestors about giving? Were you taught that you are worthy to receive and that your unique gifts are valued? Do you experience feelings of guilt when you

acknowledge yourself for giving? Reflection allows you time to integrate your experiences and remember the lessons that want to emerge. Remember what might seem insignificant may hold some symbol, metaphor or message that is calling your attention.

- **Awareness:** Decide that you will go through each day being open to opportunities to give. Take action, and be mindful of what comes up for you emotionally. Does it feel hard or easy to give? Can you notice why you are having certain feelings? Is your desire to offer this gift connected to an experience that you remember from your past? Was there some resistance to taking action or resentment after the give?

- **Service:** Try your best to approach offering each gift from an authentic desire to be of service to others. Take note of the times you go out of your way to help another person. What touched you about the person that compelled you to want to give? Are the traits that attracted you to the person somehow mirroring your own experience of life?

- **Surprises:** Approach this ritual with a willingness to be curious and surprised. Don't go in assuming that you will learn something specific, solve a problem or have an earth-moving experience. Instead, notice what surprises you about your give each day. Did you get an unexpected reaction from the recipient of your gift? Did extending yourself to another person bring up emotions you didn't anticipate? Did you receive something surprising in return?

- **Receiving:** When you give, it opens space for you to receive. Plus, saying "yes" to the gifts that are offered allows you to feel the joy of giving. Each day, notice if your heart feels open or constricted when you receive an offering from another person. Can you easily accept their gift with gratitude? Do you feel deserving of the gift? Do you give yourself permission to receive with an open heart?

- **Nonattachment:** Give your gifts with an open heart, without any expectations about what you might want to receive in return. In fact, try this: What if you were to give away something that you feel you could never part with? It could be a material thing, or perhaps a deeply held belief, behavior, or way of thinking that you feel isn't serving you anymore. Try this at least once over your 29 Days and take notice of changes you see in your life in upcoming months.

Here are a few more suggestions that should help you enjoy your 29-Day Giving Challenge:

- Set a date to begin your 29-Day Giving Challenge so that you may begin with intention.
- Start Day 1 with a short meditation about your purpose in doing this exercise. Be clear. If your intentions are vague or the energy is half-hearted, your experience will mirror that.
- Consider beginning each day of your challenge with a meditation and write out an affirmation statement for your day. Examples include:

  ~ Today I give with love.
  ~ Today I give with gratitude.
  ~ Today I give with patience.
  ~ Today I give with joy.
  ~ Today I give with abundance.

- Your gifts can be anything offered to anyone—spare change, cans of soup, your time, kind words or thoughts. Anything you mindfully offer to another person "counts." That said, watch out for gives that are coming from the following places within yourself because you will likely feel drained when giving from this space:

  ~ *The Bartering Give:* If I give, I am good and I will be rewarded.
  ~ *The Obligated Give:* I have to give because it's expected of me.
  ~ *The Guilty Give:* If I don't give I will have bad karma.
  ~ *The Begrudging Give:* He's got new shoes on, he can't need money that badly.
  ~ *The Resentful Give:* I suppose I better give because it's Day 15, even though I just spent $300 on new brakes for my car.

- Give at least once a day for 29 consecutive days so that the energy around the ritual gathers momentum. If you do not give one day, I suggest starting again at Day 1 to release the energy and allow it to build again. If this is too much for you, just pick up the next day where you left off. The important thing is not to quit.

There is a beautiful philosophy from South Africa, my own homeland, called *Ubuntu.* Simply, it means, "humanity to others." As Reverend Desmond Tutu says, "My humanity is inextricably bound up in yours." Even if we have a little, and we share our gifts with other human beings, our own experience of abundance and our sense of humanity are all multiplied exponentially. In the spirit of Ubuntu, reach inside and find the courage to give and I trust you will be thrilled with the transformation you experience. I wish you well on your 29 Gifts journey.

May the ancestors bless and protect you always.

Mbali Creazzo

Join the 29 Gifts Movement

You can take part in the 29-Day Giving Challenge by signing up at www.29Gifts.org. Any endeavor undertaken in connection with others has great transformative power. As Mbali always says, "Healing doesn't happen in a vacuum. It occurs through our interactions with other people."

On the website, you'll find several tools and resources to help you use your 29-Day Giving Challenge as a practice in mindfulness, including a personal giving blog, downloadable 29-day giving calendar, free gift cards, and more. Keep track of your gifts, make notes about what you receive, and interact with others in the community forums to make friends all over the world.

I hope you'll join the movement at www.29Gifts.org and share some of your favorite giving stories. Together, we'll raise our collective voices to spread positive energy and create a worldwide revival of the giving spirit.

Cami

Acknowledgments

There are many healers who have helped me stay on my feet and cope with the health challenges I've been gifted with in this lifetime. To all of you, I extend sincere thanks. Deep gratitude goes out to these special people: Mbali Creazzo, Angel Stork, Charna Cassell, Blair Drummond, Darshana Weill, Dr. Eric Rubin, Lori Del Mar, Beth Osmer, Miria Toveg, Dr. Jane Kim, Eric Small, Nell Waters, Pamela Rosin, Savrah Kramer, Karen Roberts, Shane Young, Erika Leder, Grace Ko, Dr. Peter Hahn, Dr. Norman Namerow, Dr. Lee Sadja, the fabulous nurses and staff at UCLA and Resnick Neuropsych hospitals, and Dr. Ari Greene and the wonderful staff at the UCSF MS Center. Thanks also to the great people at the MS Society, both the national and Southern California offices, who have provided me with support and assistance.

I also wish to thank my agent, Rita Rosenkranz, and editor, Katie McHugh, for seeing the spark in my story and helping to fan the flames to turn it into a book. Huge thanks to development editor Linda Carbone, who magically showed up during the rewriting stage and helped me deliver this baby. Much gratitude to my friends Reece Johnson, Mary Beave, Tyna Werner, Natasha Soudek, and Mark Atherlay who answered SOS calls for writing and editing help. Since I am physically capable of spending only two hours a day at the computer, the monolithic task of telling this story would not have happened without all of you. Eve Wong and Kate Prentiss are the visual geniuses behind the 29 Gifts brand and website; without your creative vision and design flair we would be nowhere.

I don't think I could have made it through the first year after my diagnosis if it weren't for the rock-solid support of my husband, Mark Atherlay, my parents, sisters, and my extended family members—and of course my close-knit circle of friends who are all like family to me. Thank you for laughing and crying with me through all of this.

Most important, thank you to each and every member of the www.29Gifts.org Community who has shared their gifts with the world. I'm so grateful for your commitment to help revive the giving spirit in the world. Special thanks go out to Erin Monahan, our www.29Gifts.org Community Manager, and the wonderful team of volunteers who keep our website running. Many have provided service to our community. This project would not have taken root to grow without your support. And of course much gratitude goes out to Mbali Creazzo and the many other spiritual teachers and mentors who have helped me along my path.

About Mbali Creazzo

My journey originated in South Africa, where I was born, and continued in London, where I became a massage therapist. This work was a catalyst for my own healing and exploration into what it means to heal. This interest took me to a master's degree at the age of 46, where I was educated to postgraduate level in Integrative Medicine, the practice of combining alternative medicine with Western techniques. I moved to the United States in 1998. I was fortunate enough to be invited to join a very progressive medical establishment in San Francisco, later named the healthiest hospital in the United States because of its Integrative Medicine model. I devised an integrative bodywork program sought by other hospitals all over the country, and I was core in the creating of the Transformative Education curriculum. In that time, my work with students and patients awakened me to the concept of the uniqueness of healing. Why did the same illness or the same traumatic event impact people in such different ways?

I met my spiritual teachers in the Bay Area—*spirituality,* for me, being defined as connection to all the worlds: inner, outer, other, and natural. From Malidoma Patrice Some, a prominent African shaman and educator, I learned that the power of connection to my ancestors and ritual are important tools for healing. From Michael Meade, storyteller, psychologist, tribalist, and mythologist, I learned about the power of telling one's story as a diagnostic tool. He also embraces ritual and the arts as a path to healing. Angeles Arrien, anthropologist and leadership consultant, tapped into my indigenous soul, and my appetite was tantalized by indigenous world practices to healing. Jett Psaris, psychologist, helped me to heal my relationships and taught me much about the art of working with group dynamics. Recently, my path has taken me into HIV and AIDS counseling and education, where I am blessed to work in harm reduction for homeless people and substance addicts.

I am deeply grateful to all who have crossed my path and allowed me to delve into my exploration of this important task—healing ourselves so we can serve others. Today I am a diviner, transformative guide, teacher, and keeper of ancestral medicine. I introduce people to the concept of a connection to their ancestors as allies in this world and the importance of understanding the legacy we carry as a key to healing our own wounds.